WELCOME TO MOTHER-HOOD, BITCHES

VICTORIA EMES

WELCOME TO MOTHERHOOD, BITCHES

THE REAL GUIDE TO PREGNANCY, BIRTH AND BEYOND

HarperCollins*Publishers*

HarperCollins*Publishers*
1 London Bridge Street
London SE1 9GF

www.harpercollins.co.uk

HarperCollins*Publishers*
1st Floor, Watermarque Building, Ringsend Road
Dublin 4, Ireland

First published by HarperCollins*Publishers* 2022

1 3 5 7 9 10 8 6 4 2

A catalogue record of this book is
available from the British Library

HB ISBN 978-0-00-845355-8
TPB ISBN 978-0-00852076-2

Printed and bound in the UK using 100%
renewable electricity at CPI Group (UK) Ltd

MIX
Paper from
responsible sources
FSC
www.fsc.org
FSC™ C007454

The advice and information in this book should be used to supplement
rather than replace the advice of your doctor or another trained health
professional. If you know or suspect you have a health problem, it is
recommended that you seek your doctor's advice before embarking on
any medical programme or treatment. All efforts have been made to
assure the accuracy of the information contained in this book as of the
date of publication. This publisher and the author disclaim liability for
any medical outcomes that may occur as a result of applying the
methods suggested in this book.

For Rob, Oliver and Edith

CONTENTS

INTRODUCTION

Hello, bitches, it's so lovely to meet you. I'm assuming you've picked up this book because you're curious about having kids, you're currently up the duff, or you're stumbling through the early days of parenthood with a mattress-sized sanitary towel between your legs and wondering what the hell has just happened. That, or you're killing time in WHSmith, waiting for your flight to Ibiza. You lucky bastard. Either way, I'm going to take a wild guess and say you're probably here because you're searching for something that most parenting books have failed to deliver: the brutal truths about early motherhood. Well, you're in luck, sister, because as the title suggests, that's exactly what I'm hoping to administer.

Some of you may already know me, while others will be wondering who the hell I am, and what authority I have to be writing a book about motherhood. Well, let me tell you, I'm no one special, or spectacular. I'm just a very average woman who happens to be a mum, and who accidentally gained a tiny ounce of recognition on the internet talking about motherhood from a frank, and hopefully funny, perspective. I'm no more of an expert or a specialist than anybody else; the insight I have gained into motherhood comes from my own lived experience of having grown, birthed and nurtured two babies, and that in itself has been quite an education. But don't worry, the information and advice shared in this book hasn't just been plucked out of my anus. It's been informed by up-to-date research alongside input from a team of experts including a midwife, a sleep consultant and a breastfeeding specialist.

From a very early age, I knew I wanted to be a mum; in fact, I was a tad obsessed about my future unborn babies. While my peers were busy role-playing being doctors, astronauts and superheroes, I was preoccupied with shoving pillows up my jumper and pretending to be pregnant, birthing my dollies out of my tiny foof and breastfeeding my plastic offspring from my milkless bee-sting nips. Nothing carried as much significance to me as the prospect of one day becoming a mum. But fast-forward thirty years of pining over random babies, blowing many many frogs to find my Prince Charming and finally arriving at a place where motherhood was in reach and – BAM! – I got pregnant, and everything I thought I knew about carrying a child, giving birth and finally having a baby of my own turned out to be a load of absolute bollocks.

See, the biggest secret of motherhood is that in reality it's actually fucking hard – yet no one seems to talk about it. Not just from the physical perspective of having to grow and carry a child for nine months and then squeeze it out of your vagina, but also the mental and emotional toil that being responsible for the life of a tiny human can involve. Despite spending my formative years trying to latch a plastic dolly on to my tits, motherhood did not come easily to me. From the outset it felt like a torrent of physical, mental and emotional headfuckery that left my body feeling like a tattered ragdoll and my mind in a permanent fog of unknowing. Becoming a mother made me feel more alone, isolated and bewildered than I have ever felt in my entire life. And all at a time when I needed support the most.

But that's where I hope this book will come in handy. Think of the next thirteen chapters as your pregnancy, birth and postpartum BFF. It's that special kind of mate that you can get outrageously drunk with, tell your deepest darkest secrets to without the fear of being judged, and who will hold your hair back reassuringly and ensure you take regular sips of water when you're violently vomiting up Jägerbombs at the end of the night. This book is that bird. Solid, sound and surprisingly practical in a crisis.

Over the course of reading this book, you will learn more about what to expect from the physical, mental and emotional onslaught of having kids, as well as exploring some of the more taboo aspects of pregnancy, birth and mothering that other parents are too embarrassed, afraid or ashamed to reveal and that, funnily enough, are never included in parenting books or antenatal classes. We'll start with *Pregnancy: there's an alien in my uterus*, where you'll discover some of the weird and wonderful ways in which carrying a baby transforms your being. Then we'll move on to some essential pre-labour tips and tricks to lube you up for birth in *Birth Preparation: Getting ready to ruin your vagina*, before tackling the main perineum-splitting event of actually having your baby in *Pre-labour, Labour* and *Pushing and delivery*. This is followed by the aftermath of having extracted a human watermelon out from your uterus in *The aftermath* and *Welcome to Babygeddon*, before moving on to the remaining chapters exploring everything from the struggles of breastfeeding, the hell of sleep deprivation, learning to love your postpartum body and navigating sex for the first time after giving birth. Then we'll round off with a little delve into feeling like an isolated loner in *Loneliness: marooned on the Island of Motherhood*.

I will use the term 'mother/mum' in this book as a catch-all for anyone – male, female or other – who is tasked with the duty of full-time childcare. However, the content is very vagina-heavy. Being a cis white woman, I am aware of my privilege and how that would have shaped my experience of pregnancy, birth and the postpartum period, but I'm hoping the information within this book will have universal appeal to every mum out there, no matter their background. It contains everything I wish I'd known before having my babies; from swollen vulvas, dinner-plate areolas, shitting in labour, the horror of postpartum haemorrhoids, losing your confidence and identity, going out of your mind from sleep deprivation, right through to salvaging a sex life when your pelvic floor feels like it's going to fall out of your vagina. Had I been prepared for all of that and the rest, the journey into motherhood might not have felt like such a massive kick to the vag.

So let's crack on with it, and what better place to start this journey than at the very beginning, at the moment when your baby is formed and your life changes forever – insemination, baby. Strap yourself in, bitches, it's going to be quite a ride.

2

PREGNANCY

There's an alien in my uterus

Hooray, you made it! However you got here – penis in vagina, turkey baster up the minge, eggs in a petri dish – welcome to pregnancy! Herein begins your journey to parenthood, so buckle up, babes, and let's get going.

The next nine months will no doubt be filled with a whole host of changes for you, your partner, your lifestyle and, probably most notably, your body. Although you will almost certainly not be showing yet, over the next few months you will watch in awe, and occasionally terror, as your anatomy adapts to accommodate the growing life inside you. This chapter will reveal some of the less-discussed physical and emotional changes that may not be covered at your average antenatal class – developing saucer areolas, for example; discovering your nipples have grown a beard; or the surprise of half your anal tissue exiting your bumhole.

These are just a few of the treats that pregnancy may bestow upon you.

Of course, as I will reiterate frequently throughout this book, every pregnancy, labour and baby is different, so no two experiences are necessarily going to be the same – even between your own pregnancies. Some women will sail through pregnancy with no adverse side-effects and will blossom gracefully like ethereal goddesses glowing maternal radiance and beauty. The lucky cows. But for the rest of us, it's going to be fucking shit.

I'm joking, of course (I'm not). It's not all terrible; there is something truly magical about carrying a child – from watching your stomach grow to accommodate them, to hearing baby's heartbeat for the first time and seeing them on the ultrasound, to feeling that first distinct kick. In between the nausea and the fatigue, being pregnant can feel incredible. You just have to roll with the dice that you're dealt, however vomit-fuelled or hairy nipped it may turn out, and know that the rubbish bits won't last forever. And, of course, there's a big fuck-off reward at the end of the nine months in the form of your newborn baby.

Hopefully this chapter will provide you with a little comfort in knowing that some other desperate, haem-orrhoid-ridden bitch has been through it too. Pregnancy really is a miracle when you think about it, although it might not feel that way when you're throwing up into a Sainsbury's bag for life on the District line during rush hour.

Spunkfest

Getting pregnant is the easy bit, right? You meet the person of your dreams, foolishly decide to have kids, welcome a hot load of jizz up your fallopian tubes and – hey presto – you've procreated! Simple.

Well, first time round that did indeed happen for my husband and me, with the whole business of getting up the duff taking little more than one night of inebriated steamy passion. So when it came to conceiving baby number two, I fully expected to have one dirty dingle on his dangle and my eggs would be thoroughly fertilised. But as it turns out, conception is a surprisingly complex and nuanced process, requiring very specific conditions in which to occur. In layman's terms: a bit of spunk up your minge doesn't necessarily make a baby.

Statistically speaking, 92 per cent of couples between the ages of nineteen and twenty-six will get pregnant within a year of trying if they have regular sex and don't use contraception. That percentage gradually declines as you age, and by the time a woman reaches forty-five, the chances of natural conception occurring with no medical assistance or intervention are pretty slim. And contrary to popular belief, men aren't exempt from age-related fertility issues either. Post forty, a man's sperm quality gradually decreases, making conception 30 per cent less likely for men over the age of forty compared with men under thirty. Basically, biology is an ageist cunt. But don't panic, pregnancy is still possible even with your ancient ovaries/jizz. One study found that among couples aged thirty-five to thirty-nine having regular unprotected sex, 82 per cent will conceive after one year and 90 per cent after two years – so keep boning.

I was thirty-six at the point when we began trying for my second child, so I was considered to be 'of advanced maternal age' (the bastards), and my biological clock was ticking with the alarming urgency of a detonating bomb. Each deafening tick felt like it took my ovaries one step closer to drying up, detaching and falling out of my vag like two shrivelled husks of corn. I am exaggerating; my reproductive organs were perfectly moist and juicy, but after trying for several months and failing to get pregnant, it was clear that I wasn't the fertile nymph that I had been three years previously when I cooked up my first baby.

So I began to track my cycle with the rigour of an MI5 agent on a vaginal mission to uncover the hidden secrets of my ovaries. Well, it wasn't that exciting, actually, I just did a bit of research and starting using the 'fertility awareness' method to work out my most fertile window for a bit of pum-pum action. This involved recording my basal body temperature each day, observing my vaginal discharge and feeling the position of my cervix.

Sounds sexy, doesn't it? Each morning I would stick a thermometer in my gob, record my temperature and then spend the day checking on the state of my vaginal discharge to look out for any changes in appearance or texture to indicate whether I was approaching ovulation. (It becomes like egg white when your clunge is hungry for sperm, but budding bakers beware – it makes a shocking meringue. Just ask Mary Berry.) It was the first time in my life that I'd been so intimate with my vaginal secretions. Of course, I'd seen it many times before, lurking about in my undercrackers, but I'd never scooped it out, manhandled it like putty, held it three inches from my face for a better look or presented to it my husband for inspection. He'd take one look at it and throw up into his own mouth. I felt like Slimer from *Ghostbusters*.

And feeling my cervix was like playing a game of 'what's in the bag?' but rather 'what the fuck is that in my vagina?' As you approach ovulation, your cervix rises up to the top of your vagina and becomes softer and moister. At the height of ovulation, it should feel more like your lips than your nose, but I've felt my lips and they've never felt like a plate of hot offal. Admittedly, I nobbed off the cervix fingering because I had absolutely no idea what the hell was going on up there. A few weeks of doing this and I felt much more in tune with my body and could pinpoint my exact moment of ovulation. Sex suddenly became very strategic. But our biggest problem was actually wanting to have sex in the first place. Not that we weren't still attracted to each other (I'm lying) but in all honesty, we were knackered.

At this point we were parents to a two-year-old child, and as I'm sure the majority of parents will agree, toddlers are the biggest cockblockers of all time. Most days in their company will leave you feeling like you've taken repeated kicks to the vag from a pair of size-14 Dr Martens steel-toe-capped boots. They drain every resource you have in your reserves, both physically and mentally, leaving you with very little desire or want for much else than a warm bath, a family bar of Dairy Milk, silence and an 8p.m. bedtime. Dick was most certainly not on my agenda. However, the pressure of only having this six-day window of fertility each month meant we had no choice but to do the dirty deed, knackered or not. Armoured with coffee, lube and Barry White, we accepted our spunky mission and submerged ourselves in the greatest, most regimented and functional minge marathon of all time. With a cervix pumped full of jizz and sporting a slightly chafed fanny, now began the anxious two-week wait to find out whether operation spunkfest was a success. And indeed it was. I was pregnant.

The walking dead

A lot of women will tell you that they knew as soon as they were pregnant because they 'felt different'. I've been pregnant four times in my life and was never blessed with that intuition, so in my opinion, that's a load of bollocks. The first few weeks felt much like any other; I was moody, snappy, a bit anxious, but as my husband will testify, that's just my general vibe on a day-to-day basis. It wasn't until I took a pregnancy test (or as was the case with my daughter, I recorded a continuous fortnight of high basal temperatures) that I had any indication that a tiny fertilised egg had burrowed its way into my uterus. Cue a few weeks later and suddenly the physical signs of pregnancy began to develop.

Now growing a life is hard work. As soon as your body enters incubation mode, your uterus becomes a hive of activity as your fertilised egg begins the incredible transformation from an abstract bunch of cells into an embryo and then a foetus. You don't have much to show for it at the beginning but all that biological wizardry unfolding inside you is going to feel pretty exhausting.

I actually had no idea what tiredness was before children, and pregnancy was a good indicator of what was to come once they were born. Consider it sleep-deprivation training; pregnancy is the warm-up round and having a newborn is competing in the big fight. So I'm not talking, 'Oh I stayed up to binge-watch *Tiger King* on Netflix and didn't go to sleep until 1a.m.' tired. No, I'm talking, 'Oh, I'm a host to this alien creature thing living inside me and it pretty much drains all my resources to survive, leaving me with about 1/118th of my normal levels of energy so that even wiping my own fanny after a wee feels like a massive effort. Is it OK if I just lie here for the next nine months and take a nap?' The first few months are intensely knackering, even if you spend the majority of it sitting on your arse with your face permanently buried in a giant bag of Kettle Chips. Remember – chewing is taxing, guys.

You'll be pleased to hear that the fatigue does ease up during the second trimester and, dare I say it, you may even feel energised. I mean, not enough to actually do anything with this new-found energy, but at least you'll stop feeling like a walking corpse. But don't get too excited; you hit that third trimester and – BOOM! – just like a nasty bout of herpes, fatigue will hit you straight in the vag and knock you sideways. And at that point you're carrying around a substantial extra load, so even simple activities like bending over and walking are knackering.

It goes without saying that sleep is absolutely vital during pregnancy, not only for you but also for your baby. Ironically, even though you need the rest more than ever, pregnancy can actually disrupt your normal sleeping patterns. You'll be making double the trips for those midnight tinkles as pregnancy renders your bladder about as effective as a sieve, plus your expanding width will gradually make it near-impossible to get comfortable.

Many a night I was woken by the threat of a wee trickling out my urethra on to the bedsheets or by a scarily dead arm, numbed senseless by the weight of its own mass. With my pissy hole and carpal tunnel-aggravating bingo wings, I'd have to hoist myself out of bed using a rocking motion to gain enough momentum just to sit up. My saving grace was a five-foot cushioned phallus that I kept nestled between my legs each night in the form of my trusty old friend 'Phil the penis pregnancy pillow'. God I loved Phil. He was the erection cushion of my dreams and boy did that guy know how to satisfy a pregnant woman – one wave of his polyester prick and my aching body was transported to a whole new level of ecstasy. And I didn't even have to shave my vajayjay for the pleasure. I was half tempted to whack a wig on him, draw him a face and take him out for dinner.

Phil was there day and night to keep me sated, and without him, I don't know how I would have slept. Losing out on that vital night-time rest does give you the perfect excuse to catch a little shuteye during the day. Naps are a pregnant woman's best friend, so take advantage of any down time you have and get an afternoon kip in whenever you can. Not giving you the green light to be a lazy cow or anything, regular exercise is also as important ... blah blah blah ... but take every opportunity to sleep when you can.

Pass me the bin

Morning sickness affects a whopping 80–90 per cent of pregnant women, you poor slags. If you happen to be one of the lucky 10 per cent who escape this curse, I hate you.

Symptoms can range from mild nausea through to full blown exorcist style spew-fests and can last anywhere up to fourteen to sixteen weeks into pregnancy. Despite the name, it's not exclusive to the morning and may strike at any point of the day. I was lucky enough to escape any serious prolonged vomiting, but the nausea was all-consuming, especially at work. I lost count of the number of meetings I had to leave, and the work chats I had to abruptly abandon just to find a random bin to dry retch into. Annoyingly, the knowledge that you're pregnant is unlikely to be widespread at this point, too, so explaining your mysterious disappearing act to hurl into the nearest receptacle can get interesting.

I always went with the line that I was hungover, which was perfectly plausible given my track record of strolling into work sweating Pinot Grigio from the night before. I gave a convincing performance, too, as coincidentally it wasn't that far off how I was actually feeling. Despite not having touched a drop of booze for weeks, it's an apt comparison – your body feels like it's been on a three-day bender necking shots and downing pints, but without any of the actual fun part of drinking. I got away with it for a bit until my boss pulled me aside and asked me if everything was OK because I'd been 'hungover' for twenty-eight consecutive days.

As I mentioned, morning sickness is not time-sensitive and can hit you at any point in the day. Certain foods or smells can also trigger you, which doesn't help when you possess the nostrils of an angry horse. I've always had a sensitive conk, even as a child, so getting downwind of any funky whiff invariably initiates some guttural retching. And unfortunately pregnancy just intensified my aversion to pong. I felt like that creepy perfumer fella Jean-Baptise from the novel *Perfume* (minus the murderous tendencies), with a finely tuned hooter that could detect a packet of cheese and onion crisps being opened 25 miles away. My ability to identify intricate layers of aroma with one sniff would have given Jilly Goolden a run for her money – if only I was allowed a goddamn glass of wine. This sensitivity to stench made it very difficult to keep the nausea at bay.

One night these senses were put to the ultimate test when hubs rolled in at 2a.m. after a night out with 'the lads' (the twats). As he clambered into bed next to me, my senses were immediately roused by the undeniable stench of booze. The whole room was permeated with an offensive aroma of what smelt like donor kebab meat soaked in ethanol with a shit on top. Needless to say, I was furious (and nauseous) and shouted at him to 'go sleep downstairs – you fucking stink you wanker' but alas, the booze coma was deep. So instead I spent the rest of the night lying angrily awake, and with each toxic breath that he either blew or farted in my direction I had to hold back my heaves along with the temptation to suffocate him with his own pillow. Maybe I am more like Jean-Baptise than I realised? Although no one needed that putrid funk bottled up and sold as a perfume.

It can be debilitating constantly battling with nausea and sickness, so make sure you get plenty of rest when you can and, most importantly, stay hydrated. Unfortunately, there's no hard and fast rule to keep the nausea at bay but I found eating small snacks frequently throughout the day helped – ginger biscuits, dry crackers, plain buttered toast, basically anything beige and bland worked a treat. Ginger cordial and ginger tea also helped.

But if the vomiting is persistent and you find you can't keep anything down – not even water – you must go to your GP. It could be a condition called hyperemesis gravidarum, which can quickly lead to severe dehydration and will require treatment.

Pregnancy trimesters

Pregnancy is divided into three trimesters, with each one lasting a little longer than thirteen weeks. The first month marks the beginning of the first trimester. To give you a very brief overview of what you might expect from each trimester, I've created a very simple guide:

- **First trimester** – sore tits, knackered, uncontrollable emotions, feel permanently hungover.
- **Second trimester** – slightly less sore tits, still knackered, emotions are slightly more stable but shouldn't be trusted, able to move without needing to vomit. Apparently this is the good stage ...
- **Third trimester** – tits are back to feeling sore again, beyond knackered but ironically can't sleep, about as emotionally stable as the UK economy post-Brexit, vulva like two hotdog buns, half a punnet of bum grapes hanging out of your arse.

ENJOY!

Pregosarus rex

If you own a cervix, then I'm sure at some point in your ovulating life you've experienced the joys of premenstrual mood swings. You know the ones, erratically flitting between a range of contrasting emotions within the space of a few minutes – sorrow, rage, fear, euphoria, etc. – with no real justification other than that your uterus is shredding its lining. Well, the first trimester of pregnancy can very much echo that premenstrual emotional cacophony and you may find yourself feeling very up and down, with little control over your emotions. This is perfectly normal and perfectly reasonable, given that your body is busy releasing a shedload of different hormones to nurture your baby. All that gland activity is going to mess with your equilibrium, so don't feel bad about behaving like a nutter or acting on your emotions when you are angry or sad. Cry, scream, shout, do what you need to do. You're pregnant, babe – treat it as a free pass to be an absolute cunt if you need to.

It was certainly a trying time for me or, more specifically, for my husband. One minute he would set me off crying over something sweet he'd said or done and the next minute, I was crafting a voodoo doll in his likeness to stab needles into his penis because he'd forgotten to pick me up a packet of salt and vinegar crisps on his way home. The bastard. Being pregnant can make a woman feel incredibly vulnerable, no matter how much of a confident gobshite she may appear on the surface. Hopefully your partner will be understanding and sympathetic to your needs and support you emotionally while also realising how integral those crisps are to your (their) survival.

Sharing your pregnancy news vs keeping it a secret

Personally, I've never adhered to the practice of keeping your pregnancy secret during the first twelve weeks. It's a completely subjective decision, based on your feelings and experiences, so if you want to share the news, you can. I can appreciate that if something goes wrong before that time you will be faced with sharing your sad news, but personally, having to deal with the grief of miscarriage in silence and isolation because nobody knew feels far more traumatising. I went by the rule that if I would tell them about the miscarriage, then I told them about the pregnancy. That way you have a supportive network around you if the unforeseen does happen.

McTitties

My mum has this uncanny ability to guess whenever a woman is pregnant, well before they've found out for themselves. Like some medieval sorceress, she can take one look at you and it's like she sees inside your womb. She's done it to me, my sister and various other random women over the years, but when I asked her what her mystic trick was, she replied, 'It's simple. Your tits look fucking massive.' She isn't wrong.

Having an excellent rack is one of the few perks of pregnancy. Literally. Increased hormone levels boost blood flow and cause changes in breast tissue, which can lead to some pretty impressive tit expansion. These changes can begin as early as week four. Don't be surprised if your pre-pregnancy bee stings rapidly ripen to a pair of bulging boulders and you find yourself spilling out of your normal underwear. I would recommend investing in some decent, comfortable maternity underwear to house your heaving hooters. Just go to a professional bra fitter so they can measure you properly.

I actually doubled in cup size during both pregnancies, taking me up to an impressive Jordan-esque FF. I loved them. But the downside to having hormonally pumped-up boobies was the accompanying soreness and sensitivity that came with their increased mass. They were great to look at but even a gentle stroke felt like a massive punch to the nork. Luckily this sensitivity did subside after the first trimester, but as a general rule I operated a no-touching policy, which sometimes even extended to my bra. There were days at work where I couldn't bear the discomfort of confinement any longer and would have to slyly unhook my bra at my desk for a breather. Not ideal when your boss rocks up, parks themselves directly in your tit line and decides to launch a 20-minute discussion about marketing strategy and all you can focus on is the fact that your funbags are hanging free and easy at your desk like two wayward bowling balls.

As your pregnancy progresses, you may also notice your areolas changing in both size and colour, growing larger and darker as your boobies prepare for breastfeeding. From a biological point of view, these changes supposedly occur to help your newborn locate your nipple so they can attach to feed. It's technically aiding their survival, but is it absolutely necessary to make them visible from space? There was no way my baby would be having any issues finding my monstrous mammary glands, they were like helicopter landing pads. The colour change was pretty dramatic for me, with my nips moving impressively through a colour palette of palest pink to the deepest brown. So what began as two beautiful, delicate, blush rosebuds slowly evolved into a pair of dinner plate-sized, chocolate-covered digestive biscuits. I could have inspired a new Farrow & Ball colour range: 'Colour by Udder' – six exclusive shades of pregnancy areola, from 'Flamingo Flange' to 'Mahogany Mamilla'.

To add further intrigue to the ever-evolving colour palette of my nips, at about eighteen weeks pregnant I also started to notice a distinct cheesy aroma emitting from my tits. It was subtle at first, mild and inoffensive like a Dairylea triangle, but over a couple of weeks it grew stronger and more noticeable. One day I took my bra off and was hit with the pungent hum of a mouldy udder that smelt like a packet of feta cheese left to rot at the back of the fridge. My funbags stank. I inspected my breasts and noticed that a thick scab had formed at the end of each nipple. Fear and curiosity fuelled me to grab the nearest pair of tweezers and excavate these offensive Parmesan crusts. To my relief, it was just dried milk. Not realising, I had leaked colostrum and left it to ripen like a soft French Brie. So don't be alarmed if your melons start to pong – your body is getting ready to feed your baby. Just maybe don't leave it as long as I did to investigate your cheese-like perfume, unless of course you have ambitions to set up your own artisan tit-fromagerie.

Luckily, the saucer nipples do eventually return to their former shade and shape once the baby has popped out, although they do continue to whiff throughout breastfeeding. Takes a while, mind, but have faith, they'll get there. However, I'm devastated to report that the additional bulk of your buoyant boobies is unlikely to hang around either, and your voluptuous bangers may be disappointingly deflated by approximately six months postpartum. It's like replacing hot air balloons for windsocks. But we'll get to those beauties in the Chapter 12 when we discuss body confidence.

Don't be a cunt, hands off the bump

As you've probably discovered, being visibly pregnant seems to invite all manner of unsolicited attention from the people around you. Whether it's a family member, a friend, a work colleague or even a complete stranger, having a baby bump apparently renders you public property. Expect uninvited belly rubs, casual comments about your increasing weight gain and, my favourite, random women regaling you with a full-blown minute-by-minute gory breakdown of how they almost shat out their own kidneys while giving birth. Seriously, Brenda, an in-depth description of your third-degree vaginal tear while I'm trying to do some photocopying is not what I need to hear right now.

Don't feel afraid to ask someone to stop or to shut up if what they are doing/saying makes you feel uncomfortable. It's your body and nobody has any right over it

– pregnant or not. For all those expectant mammas suffering at the wandering hands and loose mouths of thoughtless dickwads, here's a handy list of comebacks to arm yourself with in the event of a bump misjustice. Remember, ladies, we might not feel it but our pregnant bodies are beautiful. And if anyone says otherwise, they're a dick! POWER TO THE PREGGOS!

The pregnancy commentating twat:	You:
'You sure it's not twins in there?'	'Well, Brian, the wonder of ultrasound is that it allows the sonographer to see inside my womb, so if I was indeed carrying twins then I'm pretty sure it would have been picked up by now, don't you? Don't be a twat, Brian.'
'You look like you're ready to burst.'	'You look like you're ready for a punch in the face.'
'Eating for two are we?'	'What's your excuse, you fat twat?'
'Ohhh, you're small/big for XX weeks.'	'Thank you for your insightful observation, Jean, but can you please fuck off.'

Curse of the pregnancy bloat

Weight gain during pregnancy is normal and necessary, as your body requires additional nutrients for the development of the foetus and stores more fat to prepare for breastfeeding. I for one gained a whopping four and a half stone during my first pregnancy and then a slightly tamer three and a half stone with my second. I was huge, but that came as no surprise, as despite the recommendation to only eat an additional 200 calories a day from the third trimester, I ate like an absolute pig. I mean, come on, the only joy that pregnant bints have is food!

Personally, I found my expanding pregnant body a revelation. For the first time in my life I didn't have to worry about aspiring to be a size 10 or having a pert ass or a flat stomach. For someone who has always been conscious of what they eat, has exercised excessively to stay slim and has felt the pressure of conforming to an unrealistic beauty standard set by a bunch of advertising pricks, pregnancy was fucking liberating.

I ate without guilt for the first time in my life. I loved the curves and the bumps that I saw in the mirror. I felt empowered by the sheer mass of my beautiful body. All things that women have been conditioned to fear. I wore tight clothes to show off my bump and watched in awe as it grew larger and rounder with each passing month and mouthful. So, fuck feeling shit about getting bigger, girls. I mean, don't be as irresponsible around a Greggs bakery as I was, but eat the cake, screw the calories and enjoy your pregnant splendour.

Alongside my glorious bump, there were, however, a few areas of my anatomy that I wasn't quite so thrilled to see expanding. My fingers, for one, almost doubled in size, swiftly followed by my feet. My once-slim, dainty digits ballooned into ten porky chipolatas that looked and felt like overstuffed sausages fit to burst. My wedding band became increasingly tight until one day I woke up and my flesh had literally enveloped my ring, leaving me with a throbbing, engorged, purple finger that looked like an angry erection attached to my hand. Panicked by the prospect of losing a digit, I tried sliding it off but that only served to make my finger stiffy even more furious. I enlisted the help of my husband, who suggested we oil it up before pulling off the ring. I've heard that before, mate. He reached over to his bedside table, pulled out a bottle of Durex Play tingling lube and squirted it liberally on to my finger. He then proceeded to furiously wank my finger until it reached climax and shot its load (the ring) across the bed. It was like some sort of weird gender role-reversal exercise and, I have to be honest, I enjoyed it. Safe to say I didn't get a ring on my hand for the rest of my pregnancy and have since had to have said wedding band enlarged as a proportion of that bloat has never left my body. I blame Greggs.

The same applied to my feet. It was like trying to walk on two inflatable banana boats but without the fun of downing three litres of sangria and catching an STD from Demetriou the club rep before hopping on board. God that was a good holiday … Nobody warned me that feet can grow in pregnancy. Not just get bloated, but physically grow a shoe size. I went up from a size four to a size six over the course of my two pregnancies. My entire shoe collection was rendered redundant because nothing would fit my newly acquired pair of platypus beak trotters. In fact, my only regret about having children was not fully appreciating my pre-baby footwear. OK, so it's not the only regret; I've got shit loads of those, but having to give up a pair of barely worn Jimmy Choos was probably more painful than actually giving birth. I'D WORN THEM ONCE! And to add insult to injury, at seven months pregnant my gigantic feet were joined by a fetching pair of bloated cankles. Literally, there was no distinction between calf, ankle or foot, my legs just merged into two chunks of mottled, distended flesh. Beautiful.

Which brings me to the final part of my bloated pregnant anatomy and the one that took me most by surprise. Can you guess what it was? My face maybe? Or perhaps my bingo wings? No, my arse! Well, despite the answer being a strong yes to all of the above, my arse was in fact between my thighs. What the hell are you talking about? I hear you cry. Well, ladies, 80 per cent of the weight I gained felt like it had stockpiled exclusively at my flaps. My pregnant vulva was massive. It was the closest I've ever come to having a pair of balls, and much like my husband, I began sitting on the sofa at night watching TV with one hand permanently down my pants cradling my colossal cootch. Don't get the wrong idea, I wasn't flicking my bean to *Coronation Street* or anything untoward like that, but fondling it was like stroking a small furry animal. And although petting it was probably excellent for my blood pressure, I have never worked out how having a Herculean ham sandwich would be beneficial to me or the baby. What was all this extra fanny meat for? Was it providing an impenetrable muff barrier so nothing could get in or out, thus protecting the baby? Was it providing a vaginal cushion to make sitting down on my hefty arse more comfy? Having given birth vaginally, I concluded that perhaps my vulva was augmenting its own meaty crash helmet in preparation for the impact of a human head passing through its fleshy trapdoors. Well, it needn't have bothered because regardless of its puffed-up exterior, it only just survived the landing.

Chewbacca on steroids

So at this point you're probably thinking, can you just stop with the home truths about pregnancy, you twat? It sounds so unbelievably shit. Well, I'm sorry, there's still more to come. Not much; we're almost there, but let me just prepare you for a few more side-effects that you may or may not encounter – and for some of you this next one may even be a positive!

What if I told you, despite having dinner-plate areolas and hideously bloated feet, as well as vomiting on public transport, your hair might be looking and feeling the best it ever has in your entire life? Like L'Oréal mane perfection. Maybe she's born with it? Or maybe she's just pumped full of pregnancy hormones? Yes, that's right, all those extra androgens floating about your pregnant body can have mega benefits for your barnet.

Before you were pregnant, your hair grew at a rate of just over a centimetre a month and, at any one time, 90 per cent of it was growing and falling out, while the remaining 10 per cent was lying dormant in a resting phase. But pregnancy alters this natural cycle and increased oestrogen can put a higher percentage of your hair into a resting phase. So although it may appear that it's becoming thicker, what's actually happening is that not as much is falling out, making you look like you've just stepped out of a Vidal Sassoon salon. At the other extreme, it may stop growing altogether and you may experience temporary hair loss. So basically, by the end of pregnancy you'll either look like you've nicked Dolly Parton's finest weave or you'll be cast as the next Mitchell brother in *EastEnders*.

Joke! We're not talking a full-blown egghead scenario here, but don't be worried if you're suddenly pulling out handfuls of your hair. It's normal. And because those pesky androgens contain lots of testosterone, whatever hair you lose on your head may be made up for in other, random and unexpected places. There's no telling where it will grow – your belly, your back or even your toes. Having a shower will become a game of 'find the follicle'. As thrilled as I was to be blessed with the additional volume on my bonce, by about twenty weeks I began to resemble an Arctic wolf.

My belly especially took on quite a downy covering, which coupled with its bulbous expansion left it looking more like Boris Johnson's right testicle than a beautiful baby bump. This delightful hairy ballbag was accompanied by another surprise fur spurt occurring most delightfully in the bosom department. Admittedly, I'd found the odd rogue whisker pop up in the areola area before pregnancy but nothing prepared me for the full-on boob beard that I managed to amass by the end of the third trimester. But rest assured, all you hairy Marys out there, all will return to normal post-birth once those hormones stop messing with your follicles. And in the meantime, invest in a decent set of tweezers, avoid standing in direct sunlight and try not to throat punch your partner when they say, 'wow, babe, you've got whiskers'. I'm not a cat, you arsehole, I'm pregnant.

What's eating anal grape?

So this brings us to the end of our pregnancy revelations. Well, more accurately, the bottom of them, and by the bottom, I mean your anus. 'What has my bumhole got to do with having a baby? Surely it comes out of my vag not my arse?' Correct. But something altogether more spectacular than a child may birth out of your anal passage during pregnancy, potentially before or during labour.

When you're pregnant, the volume of blood circulating round your body increases by a whopping 50 per cent. At the same time, high levels of the hormone progesterone relax the walls of your blood vessels and as your baby grows, the veins below your womb (near your bum) can become twisted and swollen from the additional pressure on your pelvis. Now throw in the fact that your digestive system also slows down during pregnancy and you become more prone to constipation, that extra strain around your rectum could well take its toll on your a-hole. For 50 per cent of women this will manifest as either internal or external haemorrhoids. Welcome to the bum club, ladies.

You'll probably realise you are the proud owner of these delightful sphincter accessories when you start to feel pain, throbbing or itching in your drawers, which is frequently accompanied by bright-red blood after passing a stool. This sensation may occur randomly or you may only feel it when you're mid dump; either way, it's an insatiable irritation. I don't think I've ever identified more with a dog dragging its arse across the floor for relief than when I suffered with pregnancy piles.

Pre-pregnancy, my only knowledge of haemorrhoids was via my mum. She often complained about her piles giving her jip but I never had any real comprehension of what she was talking about. One day, when I must have been about fifteen years old, she called me into the bathroom and asked for my help. Not fully realising that what she was about to do would potentially put me into therapy for the next twenty years, I of course agreed to assist. She dropped her pants, bent over, spread her bum cheeks and said 'Can you see them? Are they bad?' Can I see them, Mum? I don't think I will ever be able to unsee them!

What I can only describe as a bunch of fleshy despondent grapes were dangling woefully out of her back passage. The poor woman looked like she was growing a vineyard out of her arse. Of course, she wasn't pregnant at this point but she is the mother to four children and there is no doubt that those anal atrocities were the direct result of bearing us kids. 'You're as white as a sheet!' she exclaimed. Yeah, no shit, Mum, I've just seen half your lower intestine hanging out of your starfish. 'Don't worry, I can pop them back in, darling,' she assured me. Pop them back in? You pop a piece of toast in the toaster, or you pop in to see your aunty for a cup of tea. How the fuck do you pop in a swollen vein that should never be on the outside to begin with?

I guess looking at her gnarled ring that day was like looking into the crystal bumhole of my own anal future. Little did I know, that years later, I'd be harbouring a similar appendage of ripe dingleberries, and would regularly find myself crouching on all fours by the toilet seat trying to manipulate the unsightly buggers back inside my body. Like mother, like daughter, they say –

but I draw the line at terrorising my offspring with my bum meat.

Now that I am quite a pile connoisseur, I have honed a bank of coping strategies that you will find below. I hope they will bring some relief to you fellow bum-grape sufferers out there.

Avoid constipation like it's the plague by:

- Staying hydrated – imagine your water bottle is filled with a crisp Pinot Grigio and DOWN IT.
- Consuming five portions of fruit and veg a day even if it means giving daily fellatio to a courgette.
- Taking a magnesium citrate supplement to keep your stools flowing out of your bum as soft as marshmallow clouds (consult your midwife before taking).
- Using a squatty potty to raise your feet off the ground when you go to the bog – you'll feel like Gollum from *The Lord of the Rings* hunched up on the toilet, but like he says, 'your ring is precious'.
- Take warm baths using Epsom salts to reduce swelling.
- Sign up to a lifetime subscription of Anusol. In fact, just become their fucking ambassador.

Are you sure it's not an alien in there?

From the moment you find out your womb is occupied, you will no doubt be obsessed with how baby is developing inside you. It's a valid preoccupation and, like many mums-to-be, you've probably already downloaded an app telling you exactly what size baby will be on a week-to-week basis. For some bizarre reason, the scale of your foetus is normally illustrated by a range of vegetables. I mean, who wants to imagine a butternut squash encased in amniotic womb juice with a side of placenta? Put me right off being a vegetarian. But other than having an ultrasound scan, there's no other way of envisioning your baby.

Generally, in a low-risk pregnancy you will only have two routine ultrasound scans during your pregnancy, one at twelve weeks and one at twenty weeks. It's both a nerve-wracking and thrilling experience seeing your baby on the screen for the first time.

During the scan, the sonographer will point out the various body parts to you and explain what is what – the legs, the arms, the head, how the heart is functioning, etc. Now if you're like me you start nodding along and saying, 'Oh wow, that's amazing!' when in reality what you're actually thinking is 'was I impregnated by Skeletor from He-man?' Don't worry if you can't work out what the hell you are looking at, that's the sonographer's job. And I'm sure, despite the confusion about the father of your child, like any proud parent, you'll take that image of your alien baby home and stick it on Facebook immediately because, yeah, it looks mental, but it's yours.

The twenty-week scan is also an opportunity to find out the gender of the baby. Some people decide to keep it as a surprise, while others, like me, decide to find out. I know some people like to find out to avoid disappointment if they've been hoping for one or the other. But having had both, I can assure you, they are equally as annoying and twattish as each other.

Props to our sonographer who announced our baby girl by zooming into her genitals and exclaiming 'She's displaying her clitoris'. Not yet out of the womb and already she was taking after her mother.

One step closer to babydom

So that's it. We've covered almost every part of your pregnant anatomy and I hope that despite potentially terrifying you to death, you also feel a little bit more prepared for some of the worst scenarios in terms of what to expect from your body. Nine months can feel like a surprisingly long time when you're in the midst of emotional Armageddon, harbouring swollen extremities and cultivating a bumper crop of Zinfandel between your bum cheeks. By the time you reach full term, your pregnant bod will be so majestically engorged that you will feel like a swollen goddess with your own fucking solar system. Face like the sun (constant hot flushes), the lactating tits of Venus, a hairy Jupiter ballbag of a belly and you all know about Uranus – that beast is other-worldly. Amazing really that the female form can transform to such incredible proportions. Let's just hope it finds its way back to Earth once the alien has landed.

Finding an antenatal class

It goes without saying that most first-time expectant parents will want to attend an antenatal class. There are always tons on offer, and if you search for classes in your local area you're bound to find an NCT, hypnobirthing or hospital antenatal class near you. Of course, it's an excellent opportunity to prepare for birth, breastfeeding and postpartum guided by professionals, but it's also an excellent opportunity to meet other pregnant women.

Why would you want to do that then? Well, this is the thing about new motherhood, it's kinda lonely. I'll go into the ins and outs of how loneliness may affect you in depth in Chapter 14, but the best thing you can do right now is get a head start and make some fellow pregnant friends. They will prove invaluable once your baby is born and will keep you company in the pits of postpartum.

3

BIRTH PREPARATION

Getting ready to ruin your vagina

The final stages of pregnancy can feel like they drag as slowly and as heavily as your distended pregnant vulva. After months and months of feeling like a human incubator, sacrificing every part of your bloated body to the pregnancy gods and losing all emotional rationality at the hands of your uterus, the payoff is finally in reach. Any day now, you will be giving birth to your baby and you probably can't bloody wait. OK, so the prospect of your cervix stretching to the diameter of a bagel isn't exactly as exciting as, say, waiting for the end of year school trip to Alton Towers or going on your first girls' holiday to the Costa del Sol at eighteen years old. But nonetheless, waiting for birth is genuinely exciting. And funnily enough, all three of those activities have a similar outcome – vaginally welcoming the digits of a total stranger. Just a shame that, this time, you won't get to neck a fishbowl of sangria or ride the log flume before getting royally fingered.

Alongside the feelings of excitement and expectancy you may also be feeling incredibly nervous and apprehensive about the reality of giving birth and the worry about something going wrong during labour. Thoughts such as, 'What if my vagina is too small to get the baby out?' 'What if I do a poo because I'm pushing so hard?' or 'What if my partner sees my flaps stretch over the baby's head like two translucent sheets of strudel pastry and never wants to have sex with me again?' In my case, the answers to these questions turned out to be: 1, it's a bucket; 2, the question shouldn't have been 'will I poo?', but 'how much will I poo'?; and 3, he did witness the terrifying spectacle of my tensile pork pie opening up like the gates of Hades, and he is still partial to poking it.

These are all completely rational fears to have when you've never pushed a baby out of your hole, and like any new experience it can feel intimidating and scary going into the unknown. Even on your second, third or fourth baby you may find yourself harbouring the same worries as you did with your first because every baby and every birth is different. Like so many aspects of pregnancy and childbirth, we cannot predetermine how our experience will unfold or the difficulties we may face. In the words of Forrest Gump's mother; life is like a box of chocolates, you never know what you're going to get. Same applies to childbirth, but swap a Cadbury's Milk Tray selection for blood, placenta and faeces and it's the perfect analogy.

However, coming to terms with this perplexing reality can prove challenging, especially for a perfectionist control freak with anxious tendencies and zero patience, like me. So over the next few pages, I'll be sharing some of the tips and tricks I used to lube up for labour, both metaphorically and literally, in a bid to feel prepared for any eventuality that was thrown my way. I'll also be solving some of the big labour-related conundrums like whether or not to shave your pubes before giving birth and how to look your partner in the eyes after they've been fist-deep in your fanny giving you a perineal massage. Essential information that is strangely omitted from the standard antenatal advice.

Of course, I can't offer you any guarantee that my suggestions for getting labour moving or my expert pube-styling tips will necessarily work for you, but hopefully this chapter will at least provide you with a welcome distraction from your massively inflated pregnant labia. Yeah, we're excited to finally meet our baby – blah blah blah – but all a girl really wants at this stage is to sit down comfortably without her vulva feeling like it's a space hopper between her legs.

Getting your vaginal zen on

The biggest and most beneficial tool I would recommend mastering pre-birth is learning how to remain calm, even when faced with stressful situations. Why the heck do I need that? You may cry. Surely the imminent destruction of my vag is more of a worry? Well, the beauty of being able to harness your inner zen in the midst of a vaginal apocalypse is the power it has over your mind and body. When you are in a relaxed, calm state your body can produce oxytocin – the key hormone responsible for signalling contractions of the womb during labour. Known as the 'love' hormone, oxytocin is integral to the production of prostaglandins, which move labour along and increase contractions even more. Stress, anxiety and fear produce adrenaline, which in turn blocks the production of oxytocin and halts the progression of labour to the point that it may even stop. Basically, we need to learn to be chilled bitches, whatever the circumstances, so our fannies open up nice and wide and allow our babies to glide out as easily and quickly as possible.

Hypnobirthing and the mindful techniques associated with this practice helped me to let go of the fear I had surrounding birth and ultimately led to a very calm, empowering birth experience where I felt totally at ease and had unwavering trust in my body. I think the term hypnobirthing can be a bit misleading, as its proximity to hypnotherapy conjures up images of Derren Brown or Paul McKenna convincing a middle-aged woman from Durham that she's a chicken on stage. It's not a case of your fanny being put into a trance but more about mastering the ability to slip into a serene state even when faced with stress-inducing circumstances. Like I said before, birth is incredibly unpredictable, but one of the things we can exert some degree of control over is how we react under pressure.

As you will find out in the next chapter, both my labours ended up being pretty straightforward, with no intervention and no pain relief. ARE YOU FUCKING MENTAL? NO PAIN RELIEF? Is probably what you are thinking, but honestly, I didn't need it. Now I'm not one of those smug twats who parades her ability to labour without drugs like a badge of honour – it doesn't make me a better person or a better mother. It was just my experience of birth, and personally the guided hypno-birthing breathing was enough to see me through the pain of each contraction. Didn't stop the little bastards tearing through my perineum and taking out half my vulva, but in all honesty, I felt like I breathed those babies out.

There are some amazing hypnobirthing books and courses out there that I urge you to research and then to begin implementing their advice as early as you can in your pregnancy. Like any skill, it takes dedication and practice to master, so you need to be committed to it.

Greased-up gammon steak

I imagine your first thought upon hearing the words 'perineal massage' will most likely be, 'Oooo, I love a good massage!' quickly followed by, 'Perineal? That sounds so exotic. Is it similar to Shiatsu?' I hate to be the bearer of bad news but this will probably be the least enjoyable or relaxing massage of your life – unless, of course, you are partial to fisting your own vagina, and if that's the case, you're in for a treat. The perineum is in fact the area of skin between your vulva and your anus – like a little fleshy (and surprisingly hairy, in my case) no man's land separating your fanny from your bumhole. Its main purpose is supporting the urogenital and gastrointestinal systems, and until now it's likely you've never even heard of it, let alone emptied a bottle of almond oil on to it and given it the full deep tissue treatment.

In theory, massaging this area gently stretches the skin and improves its elasticity, which in turn creates malleable parachute-like flaps that will gracefully deploy over your baby's head at the moment of crowning with no pain and no tearing. IN THEORY. The idea is to get both thumbs inside your vag and to gently stretch out the area using a sweeping circular motion in and out and up and down towards your anus. It's a bit like playing a vaginal hokey cokey, pulling the flesh in, out, you shake it all about – although I wouldn't suggest performing this particular version at your niece's fifth birthday party. The advice is to start the massage from about thirty-four weeks gestation and repeat daily until giving birth – which may come as quite a challenge when your bump renders all visibility and access to the area null and void. Plus, if you're anything like me, you may have totally abandoned all pubic hair maintenance by this point, so finding your fanny under that bush is the equivalent of finding a needle in an anus-shaped haystack.

Such a feat takes dedication, the dexterity of an Olympic gold-medal gymnast and total abandonment of all dignity. And as if reaching it wasn't a challenge enough, once you're there it's like trying to tenderise a greased-up gammon steak with the world's tiniest mallets.

Of course, if you're brave enough, you could enlist the help of an extra pair of hands.

This relationship milestone was crossed by my husband and me after several botched solo attempts to reach into the depths of my hairy vag alone. I broke the news to him gently over a romantic candlelit dinner with the words, 'Darling, I need you to do the bum thing I told you about and I need you to do it now.' He looked at me excitedly. 'Not that bum thing, babe, the other bum thing. You know, the one where you massage my perineum.' His excitement was quickly replaced by fear as the realisation of what 'that bum thing' meant sunk in. He took a slow and deliberate gulp of his Malbec (the lucky bastard) and accepted his mission with grace. 'If that's what you need me to do, I'll do it.'

Like two astronauts being blasted into an uncharted hemisphere, we made our way upstairs, hand in hand ready to conquer my Uranus. I slipped off my knickers, lay down on the bed, and spread my legs as wide as my gargantuan belly would allow me. With his digits suitably oiled, he moved into position right between my thighs and apprehensively began manoeuvring his thumbs slowly inside my vagina. It was immediately awkward. Neither of us knew where to look and our awkwardness was only compounded by the very audible wet squelching of my passage being pounded by his greasy fingers.

As the procedure progressed, he slowly sank further and further out of view behind my bump until all I could see was the top of his head hovering slightly below my belly button. What if my cavernous vagina sucked him in whole like some sort of tragic minge-mining disaster? I could just see the headline: MAN MISSING, SUSPECTED DEAD AFTER BECOMING TRAPPED IN WIFE'S CERVIX. At the very moment I contemplated ringing emergency services to send in snatch rescue, he emerged breathless, like a deep-sea muff diver returning to surface level after a particularly hairy dive (literally). 'I don't think I can do this,' he muttered, looking like he'd seen a ghost. I agreed. This was quite possibly the most humiliating and surreal moment of our five-year relationship. 'Me neither, mate.'

He ejected his thumbs, helped me put my keks back on and then we sat silently, side by side, staring into the distance wondering how our relationship would ever recover from him wearing me like a finger puppet.

Don't worry, it did. Just let me warn you, it's not easy looking your partner in the eye after they've manhandled your perineum like an Italian chef hand-stretching an extra-large pizza base. Brings a whole new meaning to meat feast. Oh, and for clarity, it didn't fucking work either. That's not to say it won't work for you, but it's probably going to need a bit more dedication than one brief fingering.

To shave or not to shave; that is the question

Another element of childbirth that you perhaps haven't considered until now is the very real prospect of having to showcase your fanny to a room full of strangers. Funnily enough, labour and vaginas go hand in hand, or should I say, minge in minge, so it's one of the aspects of giving birth that's kind of impossible to avoid.

With the prospect of full front-bottom exposure looming, you're probably wondering whether you need to prepare for the occasion – to trim or not to trim? Now, of course, this is a completely personal decision and there is absolutely no right or wrong answer. Do whatever makes you feel comfortable. So I decided to do a little pre-birth prep work on my pubes out of courtesy for my audience. I knew that the midwives probably wouldn't care less if my ham sandwich was looking a little furry, but for me, it just felt more dignified to give birth with a coiffured cooch. Which in retrospect was wildly naive of me, given that regardless of how neat my public hair was, my minge would still end up looking like a punched lasagne.

Not yet privy to this insider knowledge, and wanting to make a good impression, I set about tackling my hairy beast. Appearance-wise, I've always gone for a short back and sides on the foof front, achieved using hair removal cream for the sideburns and then taming the main body of wild ginger brillo pad with my husband's beard trimmer. (Soz, darling.) I managed to maintain this look for the first few months of pregnancy with no difficulty at all but as my stomach expanded, so did my bikini line. As you can imagine, reaching round to access the appropriate areas was significantly compromised by my bulbous belly and any attempts to get there would result in a cricked neck and a patchy muff as I couldn't see what I was doing.

So at approximately six months I stopped trying and gave up entirely. But fast-forward to a week before my due date and it dawned on me that my growler was looking like Chewbacca on steroids. I could have given it French braids, a pet monkey and auditioned it for the role of Pippi Longstocking, it had achieved that much growth. I felt I simply could not inflict this feral flange on the midwives, so off to the bathroom I went, stripped off completely starkers and dug out my trusty tube of Veet. At this stage my belly was so enormous that I was unable to see my feet let alone my flaps, so I decided to enlist the help of a small circular vanity mirror to provide an additional view. I popped it on the windowsill, angled it meticulously and created the perfect minge-eye-view to set about conquering my colossal clunge.

Now if you're a veteran hair-removal-cream enthusiast like me, then you're probably intimate with the pose I like to refer to as 'the crab'. It's a sort of wide-legged squat that's created by spreading your legs as far apart as possible, turning your feet outwards and ideally getting your legs at 90-degree angles. The crab creates the perfect stance to apply the hair-removal cream to the bikini line area so it can work its magic without accidentally infiltrating the main pube area and taking out the entire furry forest. Essentially, you assume the crab, slap on the cream, then hold that position until your short and curlies disintegrate (normally about three to four minutes). For a non-pregnant person, it's an incredibly simple process that requires no flexibility or strength and can be executed with the grace and dignity of a prima ballerina performing a plié. Chuck in four and a half additional stones of belly meat and the inability to see your own vagina and that grace and dignity dissolves faster than your pubic hair.

So there I was, standing in my bathroom, completely naked with the quite frankly horrifying reflection of my bristly merkin in the mirror staring back at me as I awkwardly lowered myself into the crab. Immediately, my legs started to tremble under the weight of my ungodly hulk, but I took a deep breath, unscrewed the cap of the Veet and squeezeed a large dollop into my hand. Using the mirror to guide me, I nervously began to apply the cream to the deep dark crevices between my flaps and thighs. It was a delicate operation as, despite the assistance of the mirror, my view was still very much obscured by the sheer mass of my pregnant stomach, coupled with the added confusion of having to mentally process my mirror image and work out where the fuck my hand was travelling to hit the correct area in need of defuzzing.

Mysteriously the cream kept disappearing into the vortex of my thigh creases, so I just figured that the more cream I put on, the better chance I'd have of success. Heavily Veeted, I settled into my squat with two huge white landing strips either side of my puss chops and began the countdown to removal. Within about fifteen seconds it became apparent that my quads had the strength of a wet paper towel and pretty soon my entire body was shaking like a shitting dog trying to curl a stubborn turd out of its hairy backside. Unable to maintain a static hold, I had to keep coming in and out of the stance to give my weak, feeble legs a break. What I didn't realise at the time was that each movement I made pushed the cream further and further into my crevices, but it was only when my bumhole began to tingle that I realised something had gone horribly wrong.

At this point, I grabbed the mirror, put it on the floor and squatted directly over it to get a better view of what was happening to my burning arsehole. It's an image that I think it is safe to say will forever be burnt on to my retinas. Not only was I confronted by my chubby beef curtains sprawled across the mirror but my entire anus area was covered in the hair-removal cream, pregnancy haemorrhoids included. I let out a short sharp scream and began frantically wiping away the Veet with the trowel that comes with the product. The burn had really heated up by this point and my back passage was alight with sensation. Terrified that I may actually burn off my dangle berries, I quickly jumped into the shower and jet-washed the remaining cream off my genitals and anus.

What was left was nothing short of a car crash. My muff had whole giant patches and gaps of hair missing that had been accidentally removed and my now bald undercarriage was burning brighter and angrier than a nuclear disaster. At least now I wouldn't need to worry about whether the midwives would judge me on my pubic hair, I'd just have to worry about whether they'd get radiation poisoning from my radioactive arsehole.

So my advice for conquering your colossal carpeted clunge? Enrol an assistant (preferably one who is already familiar with your bumhole), use a mirror (just don't make the mistake of squatting over it as the term 'beef curtains' will literally translate) and failing all that, fuck it right off and go *au naturel*. Who gives a shit about your bikini line when you're about to perform a miracle? And trust me, once that oxytocin is flowing and you're in the zone, the last thing you'll be stressing about is whether you've flashed your clam to the midwife. Remember, too, she's probably seen hundreds and hundreds of clams, so your hairy Mary will just disappear in a sea of unidentifiable beavers.

Writing your birth plan

As you edge closer and closer to birth, it's a good idea to start thinking about your birth plan. Now, I think 'plan' is misleading as that implies it's something you're guaranteed to stick to. First off, let's just be very clear that any birth 'plan' is going to be about as watertight as the RMS *Titanic*. You may plan to give birth in a birthing pool full of rose petals as Himalayan flute music gently coaxes your baby out of your womb, but in reality that pool may end up being filled with your turds, and to the soundtrack of cries of despair while your partner has to fish your faeces out with a colander. A more realistic term would be birth *preferences* – how you'd ideally like labour and birth to play out in your ultimate fantasy birth scenario, but also knowing full well that you may not get everything you wish for.

Writing a birth plan is now a standard exercise and forms part of your NHS antenatal paperwork. It's up to you whether you fill it out, but personally I found it an incredibly useful document to have. It's a chance to state your preferences for the environment you're giving birth in (your preferred lighting, music, general ambience), the treatment you would like to receive (I opted for no vaginal examinations during my second labour) and you can state whether you want to be offered pain relief, what type of pain relief, etc., and also your preferences post-birth (cord-clamping, skin on skin, placenta delivery, etc.).

It's also very useful in that it saves having to explain yourself several times over to the various midwives present at the birth while you're simultaneously trying to focus on the very challenging act of expelling your baby from your uterus. I used the birth preferences template from The Positive Birth Company (which you can find on their website: www.thepositivebirthcompany.co.uk), with some personal amendments, and printed it out several times to simply hand to the midwife.

Let's get this show on the road!

Once you hit thirty-seven weeks you are considered full term and could spontaneously go into labour at any given point. At this stage you are probably sick of being pregnant and are counting down the days until your body is once again your own. For the majority of women, labour will happen naturally between thirty-seven and forty-two weeks, but as you draw closer to your due date you may feel the urge to hurry things along a little. Especially if you're an impatient twat like me. Scientifically speaking, there is no solid evidence that there is anything you can do to speed up the process of going into labour – your body will do it when it's ready. However, there is anecdotal evidence to suggest that some of the holistic methods listed below may encourage spontaneous labour. And let's face it, you've got fuck all else to do, so they're worth a shot.

Move that arse

Exercise is quite possibly the last thing you feel like doing when your swollen body has reached maximum fluid-retention levels, your movement is limited by the sheer mass of your vulva and you generally feel like an overstuffed sausage. But it doesn't have to be at a Joe Wicks' level of piss-inducing, pelvic-floor failure HIIT. The simple act of just walking may help draw the baby down into your pelvis (thanks to gravity and the swaying of your hips) and the pressure of the baby on your pelvis may prime your cervix for labour. Prenatal yoga can also help to encourage baby into a good position, as well as keeping you mentally and emotionally centred and serene.

Personally, I aimed for a two-mile walk every day in the last couple of weeks and regularly practised yoga in the lead-up to birth by following pregnancy yoga YouTube videos. I found it helped to quell my anxiety, keep me calm and, most helpfully, expel the build-up of excess wind I accumulated on a daily basis. Just don't get into child's pose around strangers; it won't end well. Although you could just blame it on your chakras.

Flick the bean

The theory behind having sex to induce labour is that it's essentially a two-pronged attack on your cervix. That makes it sound like you need some sort of alien multi-bellended penis to achieve this, but actually it's as simple as having an orgasm and welcoming your partner's hot jizzy deposit up your foof.

To break it down; oxytocin is released when you climax, which as we know is imperative for giving birth. Then the sperm, which contains prostaglandins, is thought to help ripen your cervix (but not before it's ready). The two combined could potentially kick-start labour once you've reached full term. And if sperm isn't available to you, then just the orgasm part is still effective, meaning you can frigg off to your clit's content. Science has failed to back this up, but hey, what have you got to lose? You get the joy of an orgasm and if your partner has balls, he gets to spaff his load. But just like the prospect of exercising when heavily pregnant, sex may seem like such an unalluring task that you'd rather cut off your own vulva than welcome a willy into its swollen folds.

Equally you could be on the opposite end of the sexy spectrum and craving a pummelling like a climax-hungry hussy on heat. I fell into the latter camp; however, my husband was so terrified that he would 'poke the baby' that he avoided my flaps like they had the pussy plague. I reassured him that it was anatomically impossible for his shaft to get anywhere near the baby, especially with such a tiny schlong. Either way, if he was worried that his genitalia would touch the baby, had he taken into consideration that my vagina was technically on the baby's face 24/7? He wasn't convinced, but eventually I lured him into the bedroom at thirty-nine weeks with the promise that he could think about Scarlett Johansson during the act and I wouldn't be offended. What transpired was the least-arousing fifteen minutes of our sexual relationship to date. Have you ever seen a grown man try to mate with an incapacitated walrus? It wasn't pretty. God bless the hubs for navigating my blubbery blowhole and living to tell the tale. Not even Bear Grylls would have attempted that one.

Failing all access to an enzyme-spouting phallus, just go solo and give that rampant rabbit a battering. Solo sexy time was my favourite pastime during the third trimester, I was wholeheartedly committed to flicking my own bean. Although again, my physicality somewhat encumbered my wanking ability but where there's a horny pregnant bitch who needs to get off, there's a way.

Titillate your titties

How do you feel about venturing into a spot of S&M? Fancy a little nipple-twist action? Or if you're feeling really brave, how about a gentle areola electrocution? Well, if you've ever been curious about how that might feel, now is your chance to indulge! Much like an orgasm, having a little nipple twiddle releases the good shit, oxytocin, and as a result could help to bring on contractions. What you're aiming for in terms of technique is to mimic the pattern of a breastfeeding baby as closely as possible over the duration of a couple of hours. There are several tit-tantalising methods you can try; hand stimulation works well (think milking an udder), as does the TENS machine (a method of pain relief involving the use of a mild electric current), or failing those options, you could always ask your partner if they'd be willing to suck on a mouthful of your areola. I attach a warning to that last option – the image of your partner latching on to your nipple and suckling like a baby piglet may never leave you and cause irreversible damage to your relationship.

Spicy food, raspberry leaf tea and evening primrose oil

We've probably all heard the old wives' tale that eating a hot curry will get labour moving. The basic theory is this: spicy food irritates the uterine muscle, which is located next to the bowel. So if the bowel is on fire with curry, it rubs against the uterus and causes it to contract. I'm not sure if it's a coincidence or not but I ate the hottest meals of my life the night before I went into labour with both my children, so it worked for me. Unfortunately, the second time round I didn't anally deposit enough of said meal before the birth and instead had the pleasure of violently shitting out a liquid hot Vindaloo directly into my husband's hands as he waited to catch the baby. So beware, that curry could repeat on you. And on your partner.

Raspberry leaf tea was a firm favourite of mine during the last stages of pregnancy and I chugged back litres of the shit in the hope that it would 'ripen' my cervix for labour. You need to aim for between four and six cups a day, which gets pretty bloody boring pretty bloody quickly. I opted to brew six teabags in two litres of boiling water, cooled it down, stuck it in the fridge and worked my way through it like an iced tea. It tasted like a no-brand, budget-supermarket crap version of Ribena, but drinking it cold made it far more palatable.

Some studies have shown that a high dose of evening primrose oil can help the cervix soften and efface (thin out), which could trigger labour and shorter contractions. You have the option of taking this orally from thirty-eight weeks or you can get a bit saucy and take it up your minge. No joke, pop a capsule up there before bedtime and apparently your quim gobbles it up like a vaginal Alka-Seltzer. Although I can testify that my vagina did not possess the power to dissolve gelatine capsules. Guaranteed, the next day I'd wake up with random globs in my knickers and a fanny stinking like Holland & Barrett.

Castor oil

This is another old-school remedy for kick-starting labour that involves ingesting a one-time dose of 60ml of castor oil at about forty or forty-one weeks of pregnancy. The castor oil is usually mixed with another liquid, such as juice, to mask the fact that is tastes like petrol. It works similarly to spicy food, in that it aggravates the bowels and thus stimulates the cervix. I definitely would not recommend this to anyone. Despite seriously considering necking this to get my daughter out, I refrained from the castor oil cocktail in the end as my midwife friend warned me that it would make me shit and vomit so horrendously that the birth would seem enjoyable in comparison. Don't do it to your bumhole, ladies.

A word from Rob

The big day has arrived. I'm going to assume, as you are reading this, that you're not a 1950s husband in the waiting room smoking a pipe, who'll be off to the pub to celebrate when the nurse announces you have a new arrival. (If you are the expectant mum reading this and this is your partner, get rid and sort out a new birth partner ASAP!) Instead, you're going to be rolling up your sleeves and getting involved. But what can you expect if you are not planning to hang around the waiting room?

The best piece of advice I could give is to do your research and be prepared. Don't try to wing it! The birth partner needs to be able to take responsibility for decision-making and admin so the (almost) mum can focus on the whole pushing a mini human out of their hole thing. I've witnessed this feat twice; it's pretty impressive and I definitely wouldn't volunteer to do it myself. She needs to stay relaxed and super chilled, and answering questions won't keep her zen, man. So take the lead in decision-making, whether that's choosing the snacks she'd like (you need to keep her energy and fluid levels up throughout), what Spotify playlist she wants (no surprise, happy hardcore when it's time to push), timing contractions (there are apps for this) or, most importantly, fielding questions from medical professionals.

To make some of the medical decisions, you need to know her birth preferences inside and out. I found attending the hypnobirthing course really useful for this. I not only knew what she wanted but also understood the benefits and risks of potential interventions that could be offered. This really helps, so that you don't just say yes to everything without questioning why, within reason, as obviously mother and baby's health is the most important thing. (I realise some of you might have a partner who likes to control every tiny detail of life and would be more stressed giving up control, so if that's your situation, feel free to ignore my advice). Familiarise yourself with the different stages of the birth – the whole chapter on this is worth reading, and take notes. From knowing which hormones need to be released to soften the cervix and how to aid their release, to how long the gap should be between contractions so you don't end up being sent home from the hospital, all of this information is invaluable on the big day and needs to be learnt in advance.

Another big piece of advice to share is to be prepared for shit. Human excrement. Lots of it. First time round I was lucky enough that she offloaded it all into the loo before the baby made his descent. Second time round I ended up catching it fresh out of the bumhole into my open hands ... Think of it as good preparation for changing nappies.

How to prepare as a partner –
the dos and don'ts

Do
- Fulfil her every desire. She's been through nine months of physical trauma and her vulva is eight times its normal size. Least you can do is get her an extra pillow if she needs one.
- Massage her feet/legs/back/perineum without question.
- Let her cry – even if it's over spilt milk (this actually happened).
- Clean the house, do the washing, cook her dinner WITHOUT being asked.
- Penetrate her if she wants it.
- Look after her.

Don't
- Go out on the lash with your mates, come home at 6am and throw a glass of orange juice over the freshly decorated walls (this also actually happened).
- Consume any obnoxiously smelly food or beverages that may stimulate the gag reflex of a heavily pregnant woman.
- Eat noisily/breathe noisily or generally create more noise than is tolerable (this applies at any given time, pre and post pregnancy).
- Be a dick.

The end is nigh

So there we have it: your explicit guide to mentally and physically preparing yourself for the arrival of your baby. As we've discussed, the weeks leading up to birth can feel endless, so why not pass the time indulging your inner zen goddess, plaiting your pubes and spreading your perineum out like fleshy putty? All the while sipping on chilled raspberry leaf tea and bringing yourself to climax. Sounds like my ideal day, to be fair.

By the time that baby is ready to pop out, your mind and body will be so in the zone for childbirth that you might not even notice it's happening. Of course, that's ridiculous; no one escapes the pain of a dilating cervix, but the point is you'll be ready for anything. So, sit tight, get your dildo collection out and wank that baby out of you.

PRE-LABOUR

I think a poo might be coming

So this is it. D(ue) day is looming. From now on, every twitch, twinge and flutter you feel in your tummy will send your heart racing and your twat trembling in anxious anticipation of the impending arrival of your baby. At this point, the cramp that wakes you up at 2a.m. could well be the first sign that the sprog is on its way or, disappointingly, it could just be another gigantic, constipated pregnancy turd making its way through your sluggish digestive system. Either way, the chance of something exiting one of your holes ASAP is looking pretty bloody likely – there's just no real guarantee of exactly when it will happen.

As you wait for this fateful moment it's helpful to remember that your due date is just a prediction of when you might expect to go into labour rather than a definitive date for giving birth. Given that only four per cent of babies actually arrive on their predicted due date, it's better to look at it as an estimate, not a certainty. You could be a week early or you could be a week late, although in all honesty, it could be at any point on either side of those parameters too – birth is a fucking free-for-all. Whenever your baby decides to arrive, the bottom line is that the majority of them won't be doing it until they're good and ready. Babies are unpredictable little pricks like that, and they like to keep you on your toes – which, ironically, is the last thing you want right now when standing for longer than five minutes inflates your already bloated cankles to Zeppelin-balloon levels of gigantism.

Of course, being an impatient cunt like me, it's easy to become frustrated in these last few days, not knowing when or how, or sometimes even if, labour is going to start. A bit like waiting for an eBay package to arrive that you ordered months ago in the dead of night after one too many Pinots and are now desperate to get your hands on. You've no idea what's in it and every time you double-check the delivery window it just states 'whenever the hell I decide to show up, motherfucker'. Unfortunately, there's no guaranteed next-day delivery when it comes to childbirth. Unless of course you're having an elective C-section, in which case, that little peanut will be signed, sealed and delivered within a designated time slot of your choosing. Essentially, you have the Amazon Prime of giving birth.

For the rest of you, don't you worry, soon enough that baby shaped parcel will be sliding through your hairy letterbox and into your arms. So the best thing you can do is to sit tight (preferably with your legs elevated) and wait patiently for that knock, knock, knock at your cervix's door.

Now, as your baby begins to prepare for its momentous entrance, your body may start to give you some clues that labour is imminent. This chapter will elaborate on some of the physical signs you might expect to experience in the lead-up to birth; from losing your mucus plug (oh, the glamour) to developing the cleaning habits of Mrs Hinch on speed (which come in handy when you need to clear up said mucus plug), alongside some practical tips like how to distinguish between a contraction vs a massive fart brewing in your gut and what not to wear while gushing amniotic fluid in public. We'll also check in with how you might be feeling mentally in this precarious waiting stage and what you can do to stay calm and focused on the task ahead. Hopefully, by the end of this chapter you will be so in tune with your body and what to expect going into labour that when it does finally happen, you will glide through the whole process with ease and grace. OK, that last bit is bullshit, there's nothing graceful about your mucus plug falling out at the dinner table, but you get my drift.

Perception of birth

So you've done your research, you've read a library's worth of pregnancy and birth books, attended several antenatal classes, mastered the kama sutra of yoga labour poses, and generally feel pumped to shit for what may ensue when your cervix starts dilating. But despite all your knowledge and extensive preparation for this moment, there is still one burning question left unanswered: what the fuck is it going to feel like pushing a baby out my foof?

As birth looms closer and closer, the prospect of extracting a human bowling ball from such a seemingly tight hole may fill you with panic and dread. You may be worried about how intense the pain will be and how you will cope when faced with the physical feat of squeezing an unyielding bony skull through your delicate fleshy appendage. If this is your first baby, the experience and sensation of giving birth will be a complete unknown, and for the majority of women, that prospect can feel scary. It's perfectly normal to fear for yourself and for your baby. It is also normal to fear how you will cope with the enormous physiological changes and sensations in your body when they start to happen. But rather than trying to eliminate this fear, I think it is far more helpful to acknowledge it, understand where it may come from and, ultimately, don't let it dictate your experience of birth.

I do think it's useful to examine where our fear around birth stems from, as it can help us to address some of the unconscious feelings we harbour towards it. Having spoken to hundreds of women about birth, online and in person, it seems that most first-time mums worry that birth will be difficult and traumatic. But personally, that was not my experience of giving birth, far from it. It was challenging, that's for sure, but for me and thousands of other women out there, birth was in fact one of the most incredible experiences of my life.

Unfortunately, though, that's not the narrative we're predominantly exposed to. We've all been told the birth horror stories of friends and family (who, by the way, only ever share this unhelpful bullshit when you're pregnant), and have no doubt been accosted by a wizened stranger on public transport who loudly relays the moment her womb prolapsed during childbirth (again, these special moments are only ever shared with pregnant women). And don't get me started on the depiction of birth through film and TV. Unless you have given birth or been present at someone else's birth, think of how many times you've actually seen a woman in labour. Likelihood is that it's only ever been via a dramatisation on the telly – like some Hollywood bint screaming hysterically while jizzing her waters all over Hugh Grant's shoes as he prats about like a twat trying to hail a taxi. It's generally panicked and high drama, with banshee wailing and shallow panting, and invariably ends with the woman's legs akimbo as she lies on her back in stirrups, having hardly broken a sweat, let alone her perineum.

Sure, there are documentaries filmed on maternity wards which supposedly give you a 'real' insight, but even these programmes have been heavily scripted and edited to create the most compelling cinematic impact. All this makes great entertainment but it does us absolutely no favours in preparing us for what birth can really be like. It's no wonder women's vulvas baulk at the idea of giving birth when we've been fed such unrealistic bullshit.

I've promised to share my warts-and-all account of motherhood throughout this book, so let me tell you honestly, I loved giving birth. Call me a maniac, but as you will discover in my birth story, it was singlehandedly the most empowering experience of my life. Yes, it hurt. Yes, my flaps felt like they were going to explode in the midwife's face like two meat-filled fireworks – you wouldn't shit out a rock-hard 9lb turd and say, wow, that was easy! Sure, at times labour can feel pretty damn intense but remember our bodies are designed to counteract that pain with naturally occurring hormones. Our own inbuilt pain management system is pretty sophisticated, so our trusty comrade oxytocin will be working its magic alongside beta-endorphins that are released by your brain to help relieve pain. Don't let fear hinder your perception of how your own birth might play out, because you never know, you might actually enjoy it.

So how do we get to see the real deal and find a way to keep our fear in check? Labour is a private thing, and not many people want a POV of their minge broadcast across the nation while giving birth. Thankfully, there are hundreds of accounts of positive birth stories out there, in print and online, and despite the majority of us being camera shy, some brave souls have bared it all and shared their unfiltered, raw birth videos for our viewing pleasure on social media platforms like YouTube. Yep that's right, alongside the latest TikTok dance craze tutorials, pre-pubescent spotty kids playing computer games and enthusiastic crafters teaching us how to achieve the perfect cross stitch, you can also watch a baby shoot out of a vagina. The internet is a wondrous thing! So my advice? Binge-watch those homemade birth movies by searching for 'positive birth stories' (just maybe forego the popcorn if you're squeamish), continue to practise the shit out of your hypnobirthing techniques (as discussed in the previous chapter) and submerge yourself in as much positivity about birth as you can. You are strong. You are powerful and you are going to fuck that fear right up the bumhole and embrace birth. Remember, positivity = oxytocin = bagel cervix = baby out your minge. YOU'VE GOT THIS.

Where to labour: home birth vs birthing centre vs hospital

One of the many decisions you will need to make before baby arrives is where you would like to give birth. The options available for all women are:

- Home birth
- Birthing unit or centre run by midwives
- Maternity unit in hospital
- Elective C-section surgery – also in hospital

Giving birth is generally safe wherever you choose, but your needs, risks and, to some extent, where you live will most likely determine where you end up having your baby. Your doctor or midwife may recommend where they believe you should give birth based on these factors – for instance, if you're expecting twins or if your baby is lying feet first (breech), a hospital birth would be recommended. Your maternal age, your gestation and whether you're overdue will also be taken into consideration.

I've briefly covered some of the pros and cons of each option below, but it is your responsibility to research and understand the benefits and risks of every option so you can make an informed decision. And remember, you can change your mind about where you give birth at any point if you wish to.

Home birth

Birthing in the comfort of your own home, with the support of two community or home-birth midwives. They bring all the equipment needed for you to safely birth, including gas and air. This is all dropped off at your house prior to birth, ready for action.

Pros
- Getting to ruin your vagina in the safety and security of familiar surroundings.
- Your partner can stay with you throughout the entire birthing process.
- Having control of your environment, such as lighting, temperature of the room.
- There will be minimal interruptions.
- Guaranteed use of a birthing pool (you can either hire or buy these online).
- Increased likelihood of being looked after by a midwife you have got to know during your pregnancy.
- Lower likelihood of having an intervention, such as forceps or ventouse (see Chapter 6) than if you give birth in hospital.
- Getting to sleep in your own bed after delivery.
- If you're having your second baby, a planned home birth is as safe as having your baby in hospital or a midwife-led unit.
- A better chance of a VBAC (vaginal birth after Caesarean).

Cons
- Pain relief is limited. Epidurals are not available at home, but you can use gas and air, a warm bath, a

birth pool, TENS and, of course, Barry the sex-pest breath (see Chapter 5) to get through it.
- If this is your first baby, the chances of your baby having a serious medical problem (which are very low) are slightly higher than giving birth at a midwife-led unit or hospital.
- You may need to transfer to a hospital if there are complications or your labour is not progressing as well as it should be.

Midwifery units or birth centres

Midwifery units or birth centres are like a home from home and are generally more comfortable than a maternity unit in a hospital. They are either attached to hospital maternity units or completely stand-alone facilities. If they're stand-alone, they won't have immediate obstetric, neonatal or anaesthetic care. You will be supported throughout your birth by a team of midwives.

Pros
- The homely surroundings may help to make you feel more relaxed and better able to cope with labour.
- You are more likely to be looked after by the same midwife for the duration of your labour.
- A birthing pool may be available to you.
- You should have your own private room with a toilet and shower facilities.
- The unit may potentially be much nearer to your home than your local hospital.
- There's a lower likelihood of having an intervention, such as forceps or ventouse, than giving birth in hospital.
- You might be able to go straight home after the birth if you want to.

Cons

- You may need to be transferred to a hospital if there are any complications.
- In a unit that's completely separate from a hospital, you won't be able to have certain kinds of pain relief, such as an epidural.

Hospital birth

If you choose to give birth in hospital, you'll be looked after by midwives, but doctors will be available if you need their help.

Pros

- Direct access to obstetricians if your labour becomes complicated.
- Access to all the pain-relieving drugs you need.
- Direct access to specialists in newborn care (neonatologists) and a special-care baby unit.

Cons

- Being in a hospital environment may make it difficult to feel calm.
- There will probably not be access to a birthing pool.
- You are less likely to be looked after by the same midwife for the duration of your labour.
- You're more likely to have an epidural, episiotomy, or a forceps or ventouse delivery in hospital.

Elective Caesarean section

Pre-scheduled delivery via C-section at a maternity unit in the hospital. You might be advised to have a Caesarean birth if your obstetrician thinks that giving birth vaginally would put you or your baby at risk, or you might just want one.

Pros
- You don't have to endure any labour pain.
- You have a set date for delivery.
- Your vagina stays in one piece.

Cons
- Surgery comes with its own set of risks to both mother and baby.
- Recovery is much longer in comparison to a vaginal birth.
- You'll be left with scarring.

There's no way of guaranteeing where or how you end up giving birth as your circumstances at the time of going into labour or during labour are likely to dictate what happens. Like everything with labour, it's better to keep an open mind and just go with the flow rather than fixating on one place of birth, because ultimately, it doesn't really matter where you are! The focus should be getting your baby out safely.

However, it's still your human right to make your own choices about your maternity care. Legally, health professionals must respect your dignity and your freedom to make decisions about your birth and your baby and facilitate those decisions without discrimination. For in-depth information about your birthing rights, and support for getting the birth you want, I would thoroughly recommend visiting the AIMS (Association for Improvements in the Maternity Services) website, www.aims.org.uk, and arming yourself with adequate knowledge to make informed decisions.

Mrs Hinch on speed

Ever had an overwhelming compulsion to deep-clean the bathroom at 2a.m.? So much so that you slink out of bed, slip your marigolds on, dig out the plunger and get to work extracting the ten inches of matted pubic hair that's been blocking your plughole for months? No? Me neither! That is until I reached the end of my pregnancy and mysteriously developed an insatiable thirst for Zoflora and Flash wipes.

This disinfectant-fuelled desire to scrub, wipe and hose down the darkest, deepest, most filth-filled depths of your home is considered by some to be a precursor to labour, and it is commonly referred to as 'nesting'. Unsurprisingly, there is zero scientific evidence to support the theory that your sudden lust for bleach is directly aligned to the ripening of your cervix, but the anecdotal evidence from my and other women's experience would suggest that there is, however tenuous, a correlation.

From a psychological perspective, it makes logical sense to want to create a clean, tidy and ultimately safe space to welcome your baby home to. Like the mother hen instinctively preparing her surroundings for the comfort and safety of her chicks, us preggos feel the need to create a nest for our babies. But instead of using twigs and feathers, we prepare our baby's environment by deep cleaning the back of the sofa, dusting the skirting boards, washing hundreds of babygrows and making numerous trips to TK Maxx for new cushions – because as we all know, newborn babies just love bargain homewares at half their recommended retail price.

Take the last few weeks of my first pregnancy – I have always been partial to a steam mop and the smell of a freshly ducked toilet, but my compulsion to get the house 'ready' in those last few days before giving birth bordered on obsessive. No nook, cranny or crevice escaped my frenzied scrubbing, and the contents of every drawer, cupboard and room were removed, sponged down and meticulously rearranged. Much to my husband's annoyance, I also developed a totalitarian-style dictatorship over what could and could not be eaten in the house according to the level of mess his choice of food generated. For example, oranges, pears and nectarines could only be eaten in the bath, sandwiches had to be scoffed directly over the bin and god forbid he made a piece of toast! The only acceptable place to eat that crumb begetting abomination was the garden.

I followed him around constantly with the Dyson in one hand and a bottle of Dettol in the other, sucking up every speck of fluff and dust that he manged to emit into the atmosphere and spritzing everything he touched. I was possessed. And lo and behold, four days into my cleaning mania, just as I was googling plastic sofa covers and my husband was Googling symptoms of hysteria, my waters broke directly on to my freshly vaxxed carpet and labour began. This sodden moment marked the beginning of parenthood and the end of having a clean, organised house.

So if you too find yourself reaching for the Minky and stalking your partner's every move with a cordless hoover, enjoy it because it may never happen again. Kids and cleanliness are not friends but, luckily, you're going to be so busy wiping bums and placating scream-ing children for the next eighteen years that you won't have the energy to even notice, let alone clean, the various stains they deposit around the house.

Hospital bag

Wherever you plan to have your baby, including at home, make sure you have a hospital bag packed and ready to go by the time you reach thirty-seven weeks. Below are some suggestions for what to take, but remember not to go too crazy. Pack as if you're off for an overnight stay, not a two-week stint in Magaluf on your holibobs.

I've broken this down into three parts: a labour bag, a bag for baby and a recovery bag. You can pack all of these into the same large bag but make sure your labour stuff is easily accessible – maybe at the top – as you will need this first.

Labour bag

A water bottle with a straw: Labour is incredibly taxing, both mentally and physically, so even the simple act of drinking water can feel like a massive effort when you're focused on getting a bowling ball out of your body. The straw takes all thought out of the action of sipping and can be offered to you by your partner – meaning you stay adequately hydrated and can drink hands-free when you're busy hanging off the edge of the bed like your life depends on it.

Hairband: You're going to get sweaty, you're going to shout a lot and the last thing you need is your hair getting in your face and pissing you off. Whack it up in a top-knot, babe.

Lipbalm: As a self-confessed Vaseline addict, I think this is an essential item for any given occasion, legs akimbo or not. Weirdly, your lips can feel like two dried-up strips of jerky during labour, so keep them lubed up and feeling juicy with the added benefit of looking hot to boot. OK, that's a hilarious lie. You'll look like shit but at least your lips will be moist.

TENS machine: I am one of those bastards who didn't have any drugs during either of my births and I don't think I could have done it without my TENS machine. It provides pain relief using mild electrical currents and can be used to manage the pain of contractions. (See Chapter 5 for full details of how it works.) TENS machines aren't readily available in hospitals so you will have to hire one or purchase one yourself.

Maternity notes and birth preferences: Don't forget these! The midwife will ask for them as soon as you arrive in triage. Obviously, your notes contain important information regarding your health and pregnancy so far, but you'll also want your birth preferences available to all the healthcare providers who will be supporting you through labour.

Optional extras – battery-operated fairy lights and speaker/headphones: If you want to create the dimly lit birthing 'cave' as described earlier in the chapter, make sure you pack your fairy lights. They need to be battery operated because obvs, you can't light fifty candles in the hospital. I'd also recommend taking headphones with you so you can listen to your cervix-opening birth soundtrack or guided hypnobirthing tracks as you labour. Headphones allow you to fully submerge yourself in the audio and limit other auditory distractions. Preferably take wireless headphones or earbuds – no one needs a cable getting tangled in their pubes during labour. And take plenty of batteries/a charging cable so nothing runs out of power halfway through.

Baby bag

Babygrows x 8: The temptation here is to take a bazillion beautiful newborn outfits, including vests, socks, booties. You don't fucking need it, love. Save the £40 JoJo Maman Bébé number for another day. Your explosive-shitting, projectile-vomiting newborn will not appreciate it. Take the basic babygrows and NOTHING ELSE!

Nappies: Welcome to the neverending cycle of wiping a shitty arse. Pack plenty of nappies and make sure you get the right size – newborn or prem, if baby is early.

Hats x 2: Even though most hospitals are heated to 105°C and you'll be sweating rivers out your tits, babies have trouble regulating their body heat, so a little cap on their noggin helps to keep them toasty.

Large muslin cloths x 4: The muslin cloth is a new mum's BFF. Handy for cleaning up all manner of bodily fluids from vomit, spit, snot, breastmilk to tears (yours, obvs), plus it doubles up as a blanket.

Formula and bottles: If you can't breastfeed or you've decided not to, you'll need to take your own formula and sterilised bottles with you. Most formula brands provide ready prepared bottles of formula, so opt for these if you don't want the faff of having to make up bottles in hospital. You can pre-sterilise bottles at home and have them with you ready to use when needed.

Mum's recovery bag

Toiletries bag: Take whatever basic toiletries you need to survive an overnight stay. Toothbrush, toothpaste, moisturiser, etc. Trust me, you won't be following your usual beauty regime after your body feels like it's been through a mincer, so keep it simple.

Dark towel/s: Once the messy business of giving birth is done, you'll be wanting a thorough hose-down of your nether regions. Best to take your own towel for your post-labour shower, preferably a dark one as it's likely to get covered in womb batter.

Pjs or nightdress: This probably isn't the time for a sexy lace negligée. Think comfort, elasticated waistbands, breathable cotton, easy tit access for breastfeeding – if you've chosen to do so – and, most importantly, a generous-sized gusset to house your newly annihilated lower half. It's also perfectly acceptable to go home in your jammies, but if you want a change of clothes, the same rules apply. THINK OF YOUR MINGE!

Massive fuck-off knickers x 6: Again, the bigger and roomier the better. We're talking full coverage and whatever you do, make it cotton. You don't want to be hot-boxing your flappy flaps in polyester.

Maternity pads: You're going to bleed heavily for a few days after you've given birth and a normal sanitary towel isn't fit for the job. Invest in some maternity pads or disposable maternity knickers. It'll feel like you've got an IKEA mattress between your legs, but all that extra wadding makes sitting down on your sore flaps just a tad more bearable.

A new vagina: Joke! You'll feel like you need a new one, but don't worry, the undercarriage carnage doesn't last forever.

Is it a baby or a blow-off?

Approaching the onset of labour, you will no doubt be hyper aware of every tiny flutter, cramp or spasm your uterus makes as you eagerly await the first signs that baby is on its way. Confusingly, stirrings in your mid-section may be happening several times a day at this point down to a delightful combination of pregnancy constipation, chronic heartburn, trapped wind and your bladder feeling like it's being continuously choked in a vice. And that's not to mention the added confusion of experiencing false contractions (aka Braxton Hicks) alongside everything else going on in your overactive belly. So how the hell do you distinguish between the sensation of needing a giant shit, a fake contraction or a baby genuinely deciding it's time to vacate your uterus?

Don't worry, I'm here to help you! First and foremost, keep yourself regular in these last few days by following the constipation-relieving tips in Chapter 2. This rules out a turd backlog creating any discomfort in your guts and tricking you into believing the bum sausage nestling up your back passage is actually a baby. Like the time I was convinced I'd gone into labour and was ready to call the midwife when it dawned on me that I'd eaten an entire baguette as a snack and consequently hadn't done a poo for two days. Braxton Hicks, however, are not as easy to eliminate.

Despite sounding like the name of an American jock who's the heartthrob of high school and likes to finger girls behind the bike shed, Braxton Hicks are actually practice uterine contractions that occur throughout your pregnancy to prepare your body for birth. They are a very normal part of pregnancy and begin at approximately seven weeks' gestation, although most women won't be aware that they are happening until the second and third trimesters. Like real labour contractions, during Braxton Hicks the muscles tighten in your womb, your stomach hardens and you may experience period-like cramping or discomfort.

This can be rather bewildering when labour is imminent, as working out the difference between a false and a real contraction is like trying to identify Phil and Grant Mitchell in a line up. They look pretty similar and definitely display the same characteristics, but only one of them is going to end up punching you in the Queen Vic.

So having never experienced the throes of a contraction, when do you know if it's the real deal or not? Well, here are a few questions to ask yourself to help you tell the two apart.

How often are the contractions? Braxton Hicks are as irregular as your pregnancy bowel movements and do not get closer together over time. You may experience just the one or have several over the space of a few hours. Unlike true labour contractions that come at regular intervals and get closer and closer together, Braxton Hicks only culminate in frustration and rage as opposed to a baby shooting out of your vagina.

How long are the contractions? A bit like your pregnancy hormones, Braxton Hicks are not only irregular, they are also wildly unpredictable. They may last less than thirty seconds or up to two minutes (which is coincidentally how long it took my husband to impregnate me) whereas true labour contractions last for between thirty seconds and less than ninety seconds and become longer over time.

How strong are the contractions? Braxton Hicks contractions are usually weak, feel similar to period pains and either stay at the same intensity or become weaker and then disappear. True labour contractions begin similarly to Braxton Hicks, feeling akin to period pain but get stronger and stronger over time until the pain makes you question your life decisions and you vow never to welcome semen into your cervix again.

Where are the contractions? Braxton Hicks contractions are often only felt in the front of the abdomen or in one specific area. True labour contractions start in the mid-back and wrap around the abdomen towards the midline and eventually take over every inch of your entire body, until it feels like your eyeballs are giving birth as well as your vagina.

Do the contractions change with movement? Braxton Hicks contractions may stop entirely with a change in activity level or movement, whereas true labour contractions may become stronger when you change position. You can test this out by attempting a jumping jack during a contraction – if it feels like you're going to shit out your uterus, you're probably in labour (please don't actually test this out).

Frustratingly, I experienced the pièce de résistance of Braxton Hicks with my second child which manifested as a fortnight of on-and-off false labour. I'd be awoken every night between midnight and 4a.m. and spend several hours pacing the house with intermittent cramping that, despite feeling like genuine contractions, would slowly fade and then dissipate to nothing. The first few times it happened I jumped out of bed, excited and nervous that the real deal was finally kicking off, whacked on my hypnobirthing guided meditation and then waited expectantly for the next contraction to hit my body. But like every man I dated in my twenties, they were sporadic and unpredictable and never amounted to anything beyond irritation and disappointment.

Then one night the cramping was accompanied by the sensation of warm liquid gently trickling out between my flaps on to the bedsheets. This is it! I thought. Finally, it's happening! Having experienced my waters breaking pre-labour with my first child, I wasn't shocked to wake up in a pool of my own juices. I was convinced this meant the contractions I was experiencing must be genuine. However, as I removed my sodden pyjamas and made the transfer of said soiled garments to the washing basket, I was hit by the distinct whiff of ammonia. A thorough sniff of the mattress concluded that my fanny excretion was not amniotic fluid but the effect of drinking a pint of squash too close to bedtime. Yep, my heavily compressed bladder had simply overflowed and I'd wet the bed. To be fair, it wasn't the first time my husband had woken up in a pool of my piss and probably not the last.

This whole ordeal went on for two long exhausting weeks, and in the end, for my sanity I decided to try my best to ignore it and go back to sleep. It was very discouraging, but if you too experience prolonged false labour, just rest assured that it's normal. Of course, if you're worried, speak to your midwife. And while it may not mean that you're going to meet your baby in the next few hours (or in my case, several days) experiencing prolonged false labour does mean that your body is getting ready for real labour, prepping for the process that's going to bring your baby to you. And ultimately that's a good thing.

If you're still unclear as to whether or not your contractions are real or false, the remainder of this chapter may help to give you some further clarity. Read on to discover some of the other wondrous clues that your body may give you to indicate that shit is about to go down.

What happens when your baby is a stubborn prick – aka overdue

So what happens if you reach full term and there's absolutely no sign of your baby making their grand entrance? What then? In most circumstances, you don't have to do anything. You can just wait and see what happens while silently praying for a uterine evacuation.

If there are still no signs of labour by the time you reach forty-two weeks gestation, induction will most likely be recommended. Labour induction, also known as inducing labour, is the stimulation of birth using artificial hormones before natural birth has begun. You are still within your rights to refuse induction at this stage but make sure you understand the risks that come with making that decision.

You will also be offered an induction based on your maternal age, if your waters have broken or if you or your baby have a health problem. There are a number of possible methods of induction; you may only have one of these or you could end up having them all.

Sweep

Remember the description of the vaginal examinations earlier on the chapter? Yeah, well, a sweep is pretty much along those lines too. The midwife is going to be giving your cervix a right old tickle with two of her fingers, which she'll use to stretch the cervix and sweep around the outside membranes (where the head is) to help separate the cervix. It's not comfortable, but hey, at least you can tick 'get a fisting from the NHS' off the bucket list. You can go home after this procedure.

Cervical ripening balloon catheter

Balloons? Woohoo! Is there a party? There will be in your cervix! This procedure involves a catheter (a soft silicone tube) with two balloons attached being inserted into your cervix and filled with a sterile saline (salt water) fluid, equating to about 80ml per balloon. One balloon sits inside your cervix (between baby's head and the internal part of your cervix) and one sits on the outside of the cervix in the vagina. They work by squashing your cervix open with pressure from water-filled balloons. The inflated balloons stay inside you for 24 hours. This should soften and open your cervix enough to start labour or to break the waters around your baby. After 12–24 hours they will either slide out or be removed by the midwife. You can go home after this procedure and, if you're lucky, the midwife will fashion an animal of your choice out of your discarded balloons. Only joking, but wouldn't that be wonderful?

Prostaglandin gel or pessary

This procedure involves a gel or pessary containing synthetic hormones being inserted into your vag to promote cervical ripening and encourage the onset of labour by acting on cervical collagen. What?! Collagen in my vagina? Can I have some for my dry wizened face, please? This encourages the cervix to soften and stretch in preparation for childbirth and may also stimulate uterine contractions. You will need to stay in hospital once your clunge collagen is getting busy. Side-effects can include nausea, vomiting, diarrhoea and fever – so, basically, every hangover you've ever had post thirty.

Syntocinon

Syntocinon is a manufactured synthetic oxytocin that is given intravenously to speed up the process of labour. Like oxytocin, it stimulates the uterus and makes it contract. You may be offered Syntocinon at a later stage of labour if your progress slows down or halts, even if you haven't been induced. Contractions can come much faster and be much stronger with Syntocinon, and because it's artificial oxytocin it doesn't trigger the release of your own natural pain-relieving substances. Overall, it can make labour a lot more intense and painful than spontaneous labour.

It's important to understand what might happen to your body when labour is induced medically compared to when labour starts spontaneously, as this can have a big impact on how your labour plays out. Inducing with synthetic hormones thrusts the body into labour without the normal physiological and hormonal changes needed naturally for your body to get ready to birth. I mentioned our individual pain thresholds previously, but artificial hormones can create more intense pain and bring it on far more quickly, so even if you own an Arnold Schwarzenegger minge of steel, the likelihood is, the labour going to be more intense than labouring spontaneously.

Of course, that's not to say that every woman will experience this if induced, but it's good to be prepared if you're faced with no alternative. You can still employ all the pain-relieving strategies with your breath and move-ment and, of course, there's medicated pain relief too, if you need it.

Mucus plug vs the bloody show

As labour draws ever closer, you may notice that your vagina is secreting a lot more funky junk than usual. Having more discharge during this time is perfectly normal, so do not fear! It might look like Slimer from *Ghostbusters* has attacked your undercrackers but it's just your body preparing for birth. Many women will lose their mucus plug during this time, which has been acting as a viscid-like cork inside your cervix to prevent harmful bacteria entering the uterus. As your cervix begins to soften in preparation for birth, your mucus plug may dislodge and then – hello! – you might discover a hefty deposit of gooch goo in your knickers. This can happen weeks before labour begins, so although it's definitely one of the signs your body is getting ready, there's no need to pack your hospital bag yet.

However, if you notice an increase of discharge containing streaks of sticky, jelly-like mucus that is tinged pink or brown with blood, you can get excited! This is called the bloody show and happens as a result of the blood vessels in your cervix rupturing as it begins to efface (stretch) and dilate – a good, normal pre-labour sign that you're close to delivery.

Confusingly, the bloody show and the mucus plug are quite similar in appearance, so distinguishing between the two can be a bit like wading your way through a bucket of offal. Is it a lung? Is it a digestive tract? Or is it the inner lining of my cervix? While the bloody show is more akin to normal discharge, most commonly the mucus plug dislodges and exits as a thick, stringy, gel-like discharge that is either clear or slightly pink. It may leave as one delightful intact globule or you may lose it in parts over the course of several days.

As with everything in pregnancy and labour, no two women will present the signs of labour in the same way, but my definition of the two would be this: the mucus plug looks like something you might cough up during a bout of bronchitis and the bloody show is your bog-standard fanny batter tinged anywhere from a light blush to a radiant rose. If you experience this alongside any of the other signs of labour, such as contractions or your waters breaking, then, girl, it's showtime!

Third-trimester red flags

Once you hit the end of pregnancy, it's likely that every part of your body is going to ache. From the throb of your inflated vulva to the back pain from carrying around all that extra weight, it's near impossible to avoid feeling physically affected. But it's important to know the difference between a normal third-trimester niggle and signs of potential complications. These are some of the most common late-pregnancy warning signs that could indicate a complication:

- Vaginal bleeding that is bright red or a blood-streaked discharge.
- Vaginal leaking of amniotic fluid.
- Sudden or severe swelling in your face, hands or fingers.
- A severe headache or one that doesn't go away.
- Pain or burning when you pee or decreased wee output.
- Chills or a fever.
- Vomiting or nausea that won't go away.
- Dizziness or blurred vision.
- A sudden decrease in your baby's movement.

If you experience any of these or something else that seems unusual or worrying, don't ignore it. And never, ever feel you're wasting the midwives' time by raising a concern – even if they make you feel like you are. Your and your baby's health is of the utmost importance, so if you think something is amiss, contact your midwife and get yourself to maternity triage immediately.

Niagara minge

So let's go back to that Hugh Grant romcom I mentioned earlier. You know the one – all is calm and dandy when suddenly Hugh's pregnant love interest looks startled before furiously firing a jet stream of amniotic fluid out of her vag. Panic ensues and as he's incoherently bumbling around her like a prick, she defies human biology by appearing to skip the entire first and second phases of labour and immediately starts pushing. A few perfectly crafted cinematic (yet completely devoid of reality) moments later and bang, Hugh's a dad! Funnily enough, this is not how the scene plays out in real life.

Your waters can break at any point during labour or delivery but only 15 per cent of women experience their waters breaking before labour begins. It's much more common for them to break once labour is established. So despite what you've seen at the movies, it's not actually as common as you think. Having been in that percentage of pre-labour squirters with my first birth, I can also confirm that it's not nearly as dramatic. Yeah, you're going to be left with a damp patch or two, but it's nowhere near as startling as Niagara Falls spontaneously cascading between your flaps.

So what can you expect when your waters break? Well, this is certainly the moment to get excited as it's a sure sign that baby is on its way. The majority of women (about 86 per cent) will go into labour naturally within 24 hours of their waters breaking. But if things don't kick off within that time frame, then the likelihood is you'll be offered an induction. Every hospital will have their own policy regarding induction timings, but most commonly induction is recommended 48 hours after your waters have broken. However, it's still your choice whether to be induced or not, so make sure you're aware of the risks involved should you choose to wait. Either way, it's really important that you contact your midwife as soon as your waters break. They will probably give you the once over and ask you to perform a few hourly checks to make sure everything is OK. Most importantly, you need to keep an eye on the colour of the liquid exiting you. It is often clear or 'straw'-coloured; sometimes it changes to a pinky colour – and this is completely normal. HOWEVER: if you notice that the waters are green, brown or heavily bloodstained, you must contact maternity triage straight away for advice.

My waters broke at thirty-eight weeks as I was shuffling along my hallway at 6a.m. to take my morning tinkle. A strange sensation rose up through my stomach, which I initially mistook for my thimble of a bladder giving way, followed by a gush of warm liquid out of my vag that soaked through my pyjamas. In terms of volume, it was probably the equivalent of having a small glass of wine thrown out of my minge, it was odourless and was definitely more of a spurt of fluid than the sort of trickle you might expect from pissing yourself (come on, we've all been there). My contractions didn't start immediately and with the threat of induction looming (as is standard practice if labour doesn't start within 24 hours of your waters breaking) I pulled out all my hypnobirthing wankery in an attempt to get labour moving.

My husband suggested we go for a walk, so we packed ourselves off in the car to a local park to have a gentle meander. Having experienced my waters breaking once, I was under the assumption that this was it. Lo and behold, it was not. Just as we were setting off down a narrow path, surrounded by several other walkers and their dogs, I felt the same sensation of something rising up in my innards and then – wham! My uterus dumped another load of hot fanny juice directly on to the footpath. I was not prepared for this additional offloading or for the enthusiastic puppy who bounded up to us and proceeded to sniff my unsightly wet crotch like it was a rump steak at the butchers. With no change of clothes and my dignity now smeared across the face of a cocker spaniel, I had to delicately pigeon-step my way back to the car park avoiding all eye contact with the passers by while praying that the owner of said dog didn't report me to the RSPCA for psychologically scarring their pet for life.

At this point I hadn't had any contractions, but my womb had ejaculated hot liquid several times. Twelve hours later, having just crawled into bed (with a plastic sheet down, obvs) I felt the first distinct twinge of my uterus. It was happening! My baby was on his way.

Bracing for impact

Hopefully that gives you an insight into some of the tell-tale signs that your body is preparing for birth. If you suddenly find yourself reaching for the bleach, your gusset is slimier than an aroused slug and there's water being expelled from your vagina like a broken fire hydrant – it's highly likely that you're one step closer to finally meeting your baby. You may be feeling apprehensive about what is about to unfold, but don't worry, sweetheart, I've got that covered in the next couple of chapters. Remember, this is your birth, and no matter what happens in getting this baby out your uterus, you can do this. So put down the scrubbing brush, bin your soiled knickers, put your fear to one side and get ready to brace for impact.

5

LABOUR

Oh, that poo is a fucking baby!

This is it. The moment you've been waiting for. Nine months of growing an abstract bunch of cells into a fully formed human being and surviving the extraordinary physical and emotional phenomenon of pregnancy – the constant exhaustion, producing an environmentally damaging volume of methane gas on a daily basis, the hefty digestive-biscuit nipples, the ripe vineyard now hanging out of your back passage, and not forgetting your extensively engorged flaps – it's finally about to pay off. All that you've got left to do now is get the fucker out. Simple, right?

Ejecting a baby out of your uterus is no small feat, and labour is aptly named because it is exactly that – laborious. It takes blood, sweat and a shit ton of vaginal lubrication to get a baby out but, Mama, you're going to do this!

Like every pregnancy before it, every labour and delivery is different and unfortunately there is no way of predicting how yours might play out. You could shoot that baby out of your fanny like a well-oiled cannon, or equally your cervix could be a frigid bitch and refuse to move past first base until she's been thoroughly fingered by the midwife and pumped full of Syntocinon. Either way, it will quite likely be challenging and at moments even overwhelming, but it could also be one of the most incredible, empowering, awesome experiences of your life. And that is something to get excited about! Or you might hate every second of it and vow never ever to go near a penis again. Whatever the birthing gods decide to throw at you, this is the time to keep your eyes firmly on the prize. Your baby will be in your arms very very soon and how they get there is irrelevant.

Still, it's nice to have an idea of what's in store for your fanny, so the next couple of chapters aim to provide you with a general overview of the phases and stages of labour, followed by my personal experience of birthing my two children. From your first contraction through to the cervix-busting moment your baby infiltrates your vaginal canal and stretches out your perineum like a latex glove, I'm here to guide you through every vernix-covered centimetre of your baby's journey out of your puss flaps. I'll also be sharing some birthing tips and tricks that I learnt along the way, from finding the optimal birthing position, how to blow the perfect cervix-opening raspberry and what to do when you accidentally squirt hot liquid shit into your partner's hands.

But before I delve into the ins and outs of labour, I just want to reiterate again how varied birth can be. A wide range of experiences count as normal, so try not to fall into the comparison game and expect whatever happened to your best mate/next-door neighbour/ Auntie Jackie to happen to you, good or bad! Sure, we all want our babies to gently glide out of our snatches on a multicoloured rainbow. And we'd equally rather not tear open our perineums so catastrophically that our vulva needs more stitches than the Bayeux tapestry, but guys, ANYTHING can happen in labour, and as you will discover, nothing in birth is a guarantee. This goes for second, third, fourth, even fifth-time mums too (although the baby will probably just fall out with a queef by this point). So relinquish all expectations and just go with the flow. This is YOUR labour and however it turns out, it's OK.

The human biology bit

So let's start with the technical stuff. Childbirth progresses in three stages: labour, delivery of the baby and delivery of the placenta.

First up is labour, which is divided into three phases – early labour, active labour and transitional labour. During this process your cervix will thin out and dilate, transforming from a tightly closed rosebud to the open mouth of a basking shark. Amazingly, at full dilation your cervix will measure a whopping 10cm in circumference, which to put it into context is the same size as a Cadbury's Dairy Milk chocolate egg. Soz to ruin Easter, but your vag will technically have a wide-enough berth to pass 331g of delicious creamy cocoa-infused shell through its canal.

So surely passing a baby through that massive gaping hole of yours is going to be no problem, right?

Well, once you've reached optimum gash aperture, then comes the pushing and delivery stage, in which baby is expelled from your body through a sequence of ardent pushes, followed by delivery of the placenta. I say delivery but I feel 'slop' of the placenta is more accurate given the impressive breadth of your freshly stretched-out cervix.

If you give birth vaginally you will experience all phases of labour. However, if you've opted for an elective C-section then you won't experience any of the phases (you lucky bitch) or if you're taken for an emergency C-section during labour, you may miss out on one or more of those phases. I apologise in advance for potentially ruining several food sources for you, but to break it down:

Stage 1

Labour: the 'I can do this' bit graduating to the 'give me the fucking drugs' bit.

Phase 1: early – cervix dilates to the size of a Ritz cheese cracker (4–6cm); contractions are 40–50 seconds long, feel like the worst period pains you've ever had, start at anywhere from 30 minutes apart and steadily increase until they are approximately five minutes apart.

Phase 2: active – dilation continues from 4–6cm to 7–8cm. At this point your cervix has opened wide enough to accommodate an orange. Contractions are 40–60 seconds long, period pains have graduated to, well, every inch of your body, are coming 3–4 minutes apart and the resentment towards your non-labouring, pain-free partner begins to set in.

Phase 3: transitional – it's the Cadbury's Easter egg moment, people, so brace yourself. As 7–8cm becomes the full shebang of 10cm, contractions are 60–90 seconds long, about 2–3 minutes apart and you've now demanded every form of pain relief known to human-kind, plus a divorce lawyer to annul your marriage immediately.

Stage 2

Pushing and delivery: the 'I'm going to shit out a bowl-ing ball' bit to the 'my puss hole is about to explode' bit. This part feels like your insides are undergoing some form of medieval torture with a hot metal rod while your undercarriage gets blasted apart like that Mini Cooper in *The Italian Job.* 'You were only supposed to blow the bloody doors off, not three inches of my anus too!'

Stage 3

Delivery of the placenta: the 'what the hell is that alien that's just fallen out of me?' and the 'I can no longer distinguish between my vag and my anus' bit. The good news is after this bit, you're done ... until the next time you foolishly get pregnant and have to go through this entire ordeal again.

Stage 1, phase 1: early labour –
let the quimquake commence

Think of this first phase of labour as your uterine warm-up, preparing your cervix to perform its show-stopping act of the incredible Cadbury's chocolate egg transformation. This is usually the longest phase of labour but, thankfully, the least intense. If you've established that your contractions are the real deal and not just a deceptive blow off (as discussed in the previous chapter), then you can expect to dilate to 4–6cm within 2–6 hours. Although remember, normal timings vary widely, so it could be quicker than that or, quite possibly, a lot longer.

Right now your contractions will be somewhere between 40 and 50 seconds long (although they can be shorter), and spaced approximately ten minutes apart. Hopefully you'll be cruising through contractions without too much torment at this stage, so much so that you can maintain conversation throughout each one without sounding like you're straining to take a massive shit. As you edge closer to the second stage of labour, your contractions will go up a notch in the intensity stakes (the poo-strain voice will be active) and they'll become more frequent, drawing closer and closer together until reaching approximately five minutes apart.

But how will I be feeling through all of this, Victoria? Well, besides the obvious contractions, you may also experience one or all of the following:

- The backache of a woman who drank a bottle of Pinot Grigio and six Jägerbombs the night before.
- Period-like cramps (but intensify by 100).

- The chronic shits (don't complain, you'd rather get it out now than at the pushing stage, TRUST ME).
- More fanny deposits of the bloody show.
- Waters breaking (although it's more likely to happen during active labour).

And let's not forget the rollercoaster of emotions you'll probably be experiencing, too – excitement knowing that your journey to meeting your baby has finally begun, apprehension and anxiety about what may unfold and no doubt restlessness while you're waiting for labour to make headway.

But you haven't actually answered my question, Victoria, HOW THE FUCK WILL I FEEL, BITCH?! I get it. It's what every woman wants to know before giving birth. What does it actually feel like, or, more specifically, what does a contraction feel like? Well, it's a difficult one to answer because pain is subjective so we'll all experience it differently, but hey, I'll do my best!

You've probably heard all sorts of analogies relating to labour pain, with it most commonly being likened to intense period pains alongside lower-back and pelvic discomfort. Every woman is going to experience contractions differently; for some they'll be a breeze and for others, well, they invented pain relief for a reason. In an ideal world we'd all have the pain tolerance of one of those 'I didn't even realise I was in labour until a head was poking out of my chuff' chicks, but annoyingly there's no way of second-guessing how it will feel for you until it happens.

Personally, I like to think of contractions as individual micro-bodily earthquakes, or quimquakes, if you prefer. Each one starts as a gentle rumble in the pit of your uterus that rises up in a wave-like motion, tightening across your belly and back, until it feels like every fibre of your body is closing into an impenetrable clenched fist. When it reaches its peak, that tight grip is sustained for a few intense moments before the ferocity of its hold begins to subside and then slowly ebbs away, until each taut muscle unfurls with relief and the sensation disappears entirely. This is pretty much how every contraction felt throughout labour for me but at varying degrees of 'fuck my life' discomfort. On the quimquake Richter scale of pain, early labour pain stood firmly in the lower ranks of a 1–2 (inflicting minor damage) and as you have plenty of down time between each contraction, they are perfectly manageable. It's not until you reach the last phase of labour and hit a full-blown nine (all-out total destruction) that things really hot up and you fantasise about ripping your own uterus out just to abate the agony.

But here's the great thing about contractions – they don't last forever. No matter how overwhelming and consuming they are in the moment, rest assured, they will end. You've just got to find your own way of getting through each one without losing your mind or punching your partner. Of course, drugs help, but there's a lot you can do on your own without them.

One way to ride the waves of sensations and feelings while waiting for your cervix to get a wide on is to try to stay as calm as possible. This applies at every stage of birth. The calmer you are, the more of the good shit your brain will produce – oxytocin. As discussed in the previous chapters, this magic love hormone is responsible for fuelling this entire sequence of events – from driving your contractions, to opening up your cervix, to acting as natural pain relief. It's a physiological necessity to give birth and we want it spunking out of our pituitary gland like hot jizz.

So during this early stage of labour, indulge in as many oxytocin-boosting activities as possible; a gentle walk, a warm bath, a meditation, a back massage, a cheeky spot of nipple stimulation, flicking your bean – whatever gets that crucial happy hormone pumping round your veins is going to keep you chill and enable your labour to progress. You're going to be utilising every reserve of energy and stamina you possess to get this baby out of your flaps so it's really important that while you can, just RELAX.

As you'll likely be at home for this stage, you can extend this oxytocin-nurturing zen to your surround-ings, too. In an ideal world, your birth environment should be warm, safe, private, quiet and dark. Much as our ancestors would have retreated into the sanctuary of a cave to birth, we too need to feel secure and invul-nerable to birth freely – but obvs with the home comforts of central heating, fairy lights, wifi and access to medical care should we need it. Make the most of your 'cave' (i.e. home) in this early stage; turn the lights down low, switch off your phone, make sure the room is cosy and keep distracting noise to a minimum. What I'm saying is, this probably isn't the time for a living-room rave with your family and friends on Zoom with strobe lights and industrial house music, OK?

Saying that, playing music has been shown to boost oxytocin levels, so getting your jam on may actually be beneficial to labour. There's no hard-and-fast rule about which genre of music will get your juices flowing – it's completely up to you and your musical tastes and pref-erences. It's worth compiling a Spotify playlist of all your favourite tracks before the big day, so it's ready to whack on the moment your minge starts expanding. My birthing playlist consisted of pan pipes and Tibetan monks chanting, while one woman in my hypnobirthing class opted to play *The Lion King* soundtrack. Anything goes. Although personally I couldn't think of anything more vagina-shrivelling than 'Hakuna Matata' being blasted into my eardrums as my baby tore through my labia.

Creating tranquillity through your surroundings will likely fulfil your body's need to feel safe, secure and calm and you will progress through this early stage of labour with ease.

But at some point, if you're moving on to birth in a birthing centre or hospital, you will have to leave your cave and enter unfamiliar territory. Have no fear, as you can try to recreate this set-up in any location. Just make sure you pack your battery-operated fairy lights and Bluetooth speaker.

Aside from your environment, there are other simple tools available that can help you to manage the pain of contractions! Not to be that smug hippy twat again (I'm really not, I promise) but having birthed both my children without any pain relief, I found the most effective way to manage contractions from the onset of labour, was a) my physical position, and b) my breath.

Remember how TV and film has fucked up our perception of birth and the only images of labouring women we see show them on their back with their legs up in stirrups? Yeah, well you're going to want to avoid that at all costs, if possible. Imagine trying to take a massive shit lying down in bed. How's that going to feel? Natural? Easy? Effortless? NO! It's going to feel like you're pushing a poo-covered boulder up a 90-degree slope when your hands are made of jelly.

We want that baby to come DOWN your incline, not move along it horizontally, so use gravity to your advantage. Upright, kneeling, on all fours – all the positions that probably got you here in the first place – you're likely to find that these feel good during labour too. And don't be afraid to move! I'm not suggesting you pull out the Macarena, but a gentle sway or rocking of the pelvis can work wonders to alleviate pain and can actually help your baby to move into the optimum birthing position.

Now on to your breath. If you've indulged in any form of hypnobirthing you will know that breathing is one of the most effective natural pain-control mechanisms you can use during labour. The reason is two-fold. First, slow, rhythmic breathing maximises the amount of oxygen available to you and your baby – and the more oxygen you can keep supplying your body with, the better you'll feel and the more likely your labour is to progress smoothly. But also, slow breathing will stop you tensing up, which would otherwise make the pain of a contraction feel worse. OK, so some heavy breathing isn't as vagina-numbing as an epidural but honestly, the more you focus on breathing slowly and steadily, the easier it's going to be to embrace the magnitude of your quimquakes, especially as you move higher up the ranks on the fanny Richter scale of ouch.

There are different types of breath you can use during each stage of labour, but I kept things simple and used the hypnobirthing breath of four seconds in, eight seconds out throughout. I call this my Barry the sex-pest breath, because it sounds heavy and guttural and, well, a bit like it belongs to a man in a long raincoat who likes to flash his penis at unsuspecting strangers. But it does wonders to keep you focused and calm and (here comes that hippy again) literally helped me to breathe out my both my babies. If you fancy mastering Barry's breath for yourself, check out the labour tips box below for guided instructions.

Of course, you might be reading all this thinking, 'Are you actually joking you massive hippy? You can shove your fairy lights, your pan pipes and your sex-offender breath right up your lopsided labia!' Whatever you're feeling, when you notice your contractions becoming closer together, start timing them, and when they are regularly five minutes apart or less (over the course of an hour), ring the midwife. They will do a brief assessment over the phone and let you know whether it's time to go into the birthing centre/hospital. If you opted for a home birth, the midwife will make their way to your home at this point.

Pain relief, part 1: breathe it out baby

I think by now we've established that birth hurts A LOT, but just how much will vary wildly. Every individual has their own threshold of pain and what feels tolerable for one woman may feel like utter torture for another. As much as some of us would like to aim for a drug-free natural birth, sometimes that's not always possible, especially if you've been induced, as birth is experienced much more intensely. However that pain manifests, there is a range of non-medicated and medicated pain-relief available to you should you need it.

We'll start here with some unmedicated pain relief options before moving on to the harder stuff later on in this chapter.

Breath and visualisations

Your breath is an incredible tool to regulate labour pain and can be used throughout the duration of your birth. The most straightforward breath to practise is known as 4: 8 breathing (or Barry breath).

The concept is simple; as soon as a contraction starts, you inhale (either through your mouth or your nose, whatever is comfortable) for a count of four and then exhale for a count of eight. Repeat this for the duration of the contraction until it stops. It massively helps if you are guided through this by either your partner counting out loud or a meditation app that can do it for you. It's a good idea to practise this breath regularly during your pregnancy so when the time comes you can do it with little effort or concentration. As you move into the pushing stage you may find this goes out of the window, so just aim for slow, rhythmic breathing instead – again, it helps if you're guided through this to keep you focused.

For maximum breathy relief, why not throw in a bit of visualisation too? Conjuring up mental images in relation to your breathing can keep your breath steady while simultaneously deflecting your attention away from your bodily pain. Think of it as mind over minge. Doesn't matter what you imagine; your breath symbolising the ocean lapping in and out of the shore, your fanny opening up like a snake's mouth ready to regurgitate a small woodland animal – whatever takes your fancy! Again, becoming familiar with this notion and honing the skill while you're pregnant will make it much easier to practise in the midst of giving birth.

Position and movement

The second tool in your birthing pain-relief kit is your physical position. Think vertical and mobile as opposed to horizontal and stationary. Your innards need as much space as possible for the baby to move through, so maintain legs akimbo while standing, leaning over, resting on your knees or on all fours. Work with gravity and it will honestly make the pain so much more bearable than lying still on your back.

Combining your position with gentle movements such as swaying or rocking can also provide pain relief either during or between contractions – plus the motion will encourage baby to move down your pelvis into the optimum birthing position. I mean, who can resist a boogie?

Birthing ball

This giant inflatable testicle is the birthing woman's dream. You can use it to support yourself in any of the positions described above or sit on it and bounce furiously to open up your pelvis, get your baby moving down your canal and help to bring on contractions. Most, if not all, birthing suites will have one as standard.

Water

It seems like every pregnant bint and her dog want a water birth these days and there's good reason to opt for one. Water is an incredible natural pain reliever, with studies showing that women who birth in water use less epidural or spinal pain relief and have shorter labours than women who don't. The sensation of being submerged in water helps to maintain a sense of calm (which is excellent for oxytocin production) plus the extra buoyancy of your body can bring a sense of lightness and ease to your movements that give you more control over your bulbous hulk than you have when you are out of the water. It's like birthing in a giant bath, essentially, and what's not to love about that? Although watch out for potential poo and placenta floaters bobbing around – they bring a whole new meaning to a bath bomb.

Blowing raspberries

You've probably just read the title to this paragraph and thought, has she actually lost her mind?! But hear me out, this one is unconventional but surprisingly effective. I picked up this tip from all-round birthing guru and general quim queen Ina May Gaskin and her incredible book, *Ina May's Guide to Childbirth*. Ina (we're on first-name terms, yeah) states that the jaw and the pelvis are physiologically connected and the alignment and relaxation of each one deeply affects the other. So if you're tensing your jaw (which we do when we're experiencing pain), your pelvic floor is going to be tense as well – which isn't conducive to getting a baby out of your vagina.

She recommends blowing raspberries or performing 'horse lips' during contractions to effectively relax the mouth and therefore the cervix and pelvic floor, which in turn minimises pain, regulates your breath and literally keeps birth moving. We're aiming to be loose-lipped Lucys as opposed to taut Tanyas.

To perform this action, completely relax your lips (the ones on your face, not the ones in your knickers) and blow a good amount of air through your mouth, letting your lips flap together furiously, much like a horse exhaling. You will sound (and feel) utterly ridiculous but honest to god, it works, as you will discover in my birth stories.

TENS machine

Standing for the incredibly catchy Transcutaneous Electrical Nerve Stimulation, this battery-operated device fits neatly into your hand and uses localised electrical currents to interfere with the pain signals being sent to your brain. Using electricity to manage your pain may conjure images of Frankenstein being resurrected from the dead, but don't worry, you're not going to have to hook up your fanny to the mains to benefit from this nifty little machine.

To use it, you attach sticky pads, called electrodes, to the area where you need pain relief (most commonly on your lower back) which are plugged into the hand-held part of the device via a set of wires. When your contraction starts to build you simply press a button to activate the current and can adjust the intensity of the current either up or down, depending on your pain level, tolerance and where you are in your labour. It takes a couple of contractions to work out the best moment to press it for maximum relief (my moment was just after the pain had peaked) but then you'll be pressing it with the enthusiasm of a contestant on *Family Fortunes*.

Couldn't rate these enough, especially in early labour before you see a midwife – they are portable, non-invasive and you have total control over when and where they are used. Most hospitals don't have these available as standard practice, so it's worth either hiring or purchasing one for yourself. Prices start from about £25.

Stage 1, phase 2: active labour – stings like a bitch

Hopefully you've made it to the hospital/birthing centre by now (if that's your plan, or the midwife has arrived at your home, if you're home birthing), and preferably without incurring an upholstery cleaning fee for staining the backseat of your Uber driver's car with your vag juice. In fact, take a towel to sit on to prevent this very possible outcome.

Upon arrival you will be checked over (pulse, blood pressure, temperature, etc.) to make sure everything is hunky dory, and most likely offered a fingering, aka a vaginal examination (VE). The midwife will do this by inserting two fingers up your flange and having a good old poke around your cervix to ascertain its stage of dilation. They estimate how many centimetres you've reached by how wide they can spread their digits inside you, and by the time you're fully dilated they'll be able to pull the full peace sign right up your vajayjay. If you've ever had the misfortune of being roughly fingered by a fat-handed, overly enthusiastic lover with no concept of foreplay, it kind of feels like that. It is important to remember that VEs are standard NHS policy but it's up to you whether or not you want them. Personally, I found them very intrusive and uncomfortable and opted out of having them during my second labour. I would do some additional research and make an informed decision for yourself.

Contractions at this stage are now lasting longer (40–60 seconds) and coming more frequently (generally 3–4 minutes apart) as your cervix dilates to 7–8cm. You'll be pleased to hear that this phase of labour is usually shorter than the first, lasting an average of 2–3½ hours. However, you won't be so pleased to hear that contractions are now entering the 'fuck my life' zone of anguish, coming thick and fast with little time for recovery in between. But don't worry, you can ask for pain relief at this point or, if you're going *au naturel*, just continue using your breath to navigate each contraction. Like I said, it stings like a bitch, but every contraction has an end point, so just focus on getting through them one at a time.

Alongside the increasing aggravation of contractions, some other bodily delights that may be in store for you could be:

- Back pain that makes you feel like you're being repeatedly punched in the kidneys.
- Legs and thighs that ache like they've been subjected to a Joe Wicks HIIT workout three days on the trot.
- General knackeredness.
- More bloody fanny deposits.
- Your waters breaking (if you avoided spurting them earlier in the back of the taxi).
- Feeling stoned (hooray!) or in a trance-like state. This is one of the lovely side-effects of a dick-load of oxytocin coursing through your veins.

Labour can be pretty full-on at this point, leaving you little energy to focus on anything other than getting through each contraction. Physically and mentally this can be exhausting, especially if early labour took a lot longer than anticipated. You might be feeling restless and impatient, asking yourself, 'when the fuck is this bastard baby coming?' along with other questions such as, 'why did I even decide to have a baby?' and, 'please make this stop!' Whatever you're feeling, it's normal and don't worry – the finish line is in sight!

The most important thing at this stage is your comfort. If you have a hankering for something; a cold flannel for your forehead, a back rub, a gin and tonic (joke), don't hesitate to ask for it. This includes asking for pain relief if you want it. Remember to stay hydrated and continue to wee and poo as normal. Your guts may still be busy ejecting the contents of your back passage in preparation for the big push, so let it flow. Better down the bog than in the hands of your husband – although don't worry if he does end up with a palm full of poo, it's perfectly normal ... well, maybe not for him.

Maintaining that sense of calm and serenity at this stage will keep your oxytocin flowing and your cervix dilating. Depending on where you're birthing, you might not have as much control over your surroundings as you did at home. But if you can, get your birthing partner to make the necessary adjustments to temperature, lighting, sound, etc., to create a tranquil setting. Just don't start playing *The Lion King* soundtrack, or you're dead to me.

Interpret this active stage of labour quite literally and keep moving if you can. Walking around between contractions can help ease the pain and will also help your baby's head move into your pelvis ready to penetrate your canal. As contractions get closer together, you might find it difficult to keep walking but you can still shimmy those snake hips and gently rock or sway from side to side instead. Just keep experimenting with what feels good for you and utilise those optimum birthing positions referenced later in the chapter.

It's also vital to keep utilising your breath, so activate old Barry breath and as your contractions intensify, listen in awe as your husky pervert levels reach 'close to climax' status. You may notice some other interesting sounds emanating from your mouth at this stage too. Moaning, groaning and wailing through contractions is common, as is the awakening of your inner cow. That's right, along with the standard human noises you might expect from experiencing a high level of pain, you might also let out a cheeky moo. Don't be alarmed! It might sound like calving day in the cowshed but trust me, when the bovine emerges, you know shit is about to go down.

Pain relief, part 2: go hard to get that baby home

If you exhaust the unmedicated pain relief and need a harder hit than some raspberry lips and a massage, here are the medicated options available to you. Just make sure you've done your research and fully understand the benefits and risks of any medication you may end up taking for both you and your baby.

Paracetamol

You know what it is, you know what it does – but will it stop you from feeling your baby tear through your flaps? Probably not. Nevertheless, its purpose is to block the primary function of your brain telling you you're in pain, so popping a paracetamol pill will at least take the edge off … apparently!

Gas and air (Entonox, commonly known as laughing gas)

If labour drugs were like street drugs, gas and air would be your basic bush weed. It's not going to blow your head off but it will give you a gentle buzz and quite possibly a fit of the giggles. Many women opt to use this during birth because it's easy to use (you inhale it through a mouthpiece, which you hold) and you have total control over when and how much you take. It doesn't remove all the pain, but it can help reduce it and make it more bearable.

Every woman will experience the effects of gas and air differently, but it's likely to make you feel lightheaded and tingly. Some women liken it to the fuzziness you feel after your first glass of wine of an evening but its effects are not long-lasting, so if you decide you've had enough, it will exit your system pretty quickly.

Pethidine and similar drugs (called opioids)

Now we're stepping up a gear in terms of street-drug value, moving swiftly up the ranks to something a lot stronger in the form of morphine-like, synthetically manufactured opioids.

Wow, that sounds serious! Well, opioids mean business in terms of providing pain relief as they mimic the action of natural endorphins to block the transmission of pain signals sent by the nerves to the brain. So even though the cause of the pain may remain – i.e. your baby is still tearing you a new one – less pain is actually felt.

One woman in three finds opioid drugs such as pethidine unpleasant, as they may make you feel drowsy, dizzy, elated, depressed or spaced out – sounds like a great night out to me! I can't vouch for this personally but one of my friends said it made her feel like she'd been on a four-day bender at Glastonbury, but without any of the fun parts. It can also make you feel sick or vomit even if you've been given an anti-sickness drug alongside it.

You'll be administered pethidine via an injection into your upper thigh area by your midwife and the effects take about 20–30 minutes to kick in. One 100mg injection should give you approximately four hours of pain relief, but know that you will not be allowed to use a birthing pool for a minimum of two hours after it is administered.

Prior to the injection, your midwife will need to assess dilation of the cervix by vaginal examination – so if you're opting for a fingering-free birth (non-VE), you will have to welcome her digits to progress. If your cervix is 7–8cm dilated, pethidine is commonly advised against, as it does cross the placenta and can affect your baby's breathing. There is also evidence to suggest that breastfeeding can be affected immediately after delivery as the baby may be sleepy, and that breastfeeding can take longer to establish.

Epidural

If the bush weed and the opioids haven't quite done it for you and you're still chasing the ultimate hit in terms of labour pain relief, an epidural may be just be what you're looking for. A form of local anaesthetic administered into the epidural space in your back, it works by numbing the spinal nerves that carry the pain impulses to your brain so you don't feel anything from the waist down. It normally takes about 15 minutes to take effect and lasts as long as is needed, with additional top-ups given should they be required. Most women who have an epidural say they experienced little to no pain giving birth. Sounds ideal, right?

It might seem appealing to have a clunge that's as dead as a dodo but having no sensation below has various implications, all of which you should thoroughly research. It's important to realise that in having an epidural your mobility may be compromised physically by the anaesthetic, but also because continuous foetal monitoring and an IV are required you will be hooked up to a machine and a drip for the duration of your labour.

You may also lose your ability to feel when it's the right time to push or how hard to push and will have to be guided by the midwife. This can leave some women feeling out of control of their body and ultimately their labour, plus it can make your delivery time more drawn out while also increasing your risk of needing intervention with delivery, such as ventouse, forceps, episiotomy and an emergency C-section.

Stage 1, phase 3: transitional labour – my uterus is going to explode

Of the three phases of labour, transitional is the biggest minge ache of all. You are now entering level nine on the quimquake Richter scale of 'what the actual fuck is happening to my body?' with contractions hitting you every 2–3 minutes and lasting a whopping 60–90 seconds. That rising sensation I described earlier will rush through you at speed, hit its peak with force and maintain its grip over your body for longer and with more intensity. It's so intense, in fact, that your contractions may feel like they never really disappear and your body is in a continuous state of tension with little to zero respite between each wave. In this time your cervix will dilate the final 2–3cm to reach its showstopping maximum aperture of 10cm. The chocolate egg is in sight, people! But don't worry, this is typically the quickest part of labour, lasting on average only 15 minutes to an hour, so it'll all be over soon ... well, you've still got to push the fucker out but that'll feel like a breeze in comparison. Disclaimer – it won't be a breeze, more like the calm before the storm, but I need to give you some hope right now that you're going to get through this and everything will be OK, because it will!

Together with your level-nine quimquakes hitting hard and fast, you may also experience some or all of the following:

- Pressure in your perineum as if an eight-foot turtle head was trying to escape your anus.
- Your lower back/pelvis being forcibly prised open from the inside out.
- A case of the hot sweats that rival those of your menopausal mum.
- Suddenly feeling like you might vomit (which you may well do).
- Crampy legs that make you tremble like a shitting dog.
- Complete and utter exhaustion.

This is the bit where your emotions also turn, how do I put this politely ... batshit fucking crazy. You've likely been at this for some time now and, understandably, your stamina may be waning. You may be feeling over-whelmed, teary, irritable and maybe even a little discouraged that the baby isn't here yet. This is when the fear may sneakily creep in too; the panic of being out of control as your contractions take over your body and then the subsequent doubt over your ability to birth your baby. This is all perfectly normal and whatever your brain is currently telling you, whether that's 'I can't do this' or 'I'm not strong enough' or 'my uterus is going to explode', just trust in your body and know that soon enough this will pass and your baby will be in your arms.

Given the intensity of this phase, both emotionally and physically, all your previous efforts to stay calm and serene have probably gone up in flames along with your desire to ever have children again. Of course you can continue with your Barry breath to manage the pain, but with everything that's going on, you may temporarily lose focus and struggle to maintain a controlled breath. Don't worry if this is the case, forget about Bazza and just aim for a slow, rhythmic deep breath. I would say 'just try to relax' but I've been there twice myself and I don't want to sound like a patronising cow. No matter how finely tuned your inner zen is, the likelihood is, you'll be weeping uncontrollably, begging for every drug going and screaming at your partner to fuck off and die (it happens). Don't worry, it'll all be over in a bit and any moment now you'll hit full dilation and your baby will begin breaching your cervix.

PUSHING AND DELIVERY

Squeezing a human watermelon out of your hole

Now we're in business ladies! You've officially hit stage 2 of labour: pushing and delivery. Baby is well and truly on the move and it's time to get this fucker out of you. You'll know this is approaching as at some point in the madness of the transitional phase, there'll come a moment when you suddenly feel like the biggest shit of your life is brewing in your backside. Well, my love, there's no mistaking this time, that giant turd is in fact your baby. And guess what – it's ready to exit your vagina. Woo hoo!

Although you probably feel like you've already done ten rounds with Tyson in the ring, up until this point, it's actually been your uterus and cervix doing the hard graft with little conscious physical exertion on your part. But that's all about to change as you enter the pushing stage. That's right, it's your time to shine now, or should I say, excessively strain to the point of soiling yourself. This is the bit where you really have to put the effort in and consciously work with the rhythm of your contractions to help your body propel this baby out of your uterus. So gear up, hop back into that ring and prepare to take your final pounding. As Salt-N-Pepa said, 'p-p-p-p-p-push it real good!'

Like every stage of labour, how long this process takes varies anywhere from a few minutes to several hours, but the average delivery time is around 30–60 minutes long. Breezy girls! You've probably taken bigger shits than that! You'll be pleased to hear that your contractions should have chilled the fuck out from the transition phase and are now coming slightly further apart, every 2–5 minutes. They are still between 60–90 seconds long, but with less ferocity there's an opportunity to rest between them, so all in all, things will hopefully feel a lot less chaotic. I mean, ejecting a living thing out of your front bum is still going to take a lot of effort, but hey, let's find the positives where we can.

Other common occurrences during this stage (although you may not experience these at all if you've had an epidural, ya lucky bitch!):

- An overwhelming urge to push – much like the urgency of needing a massive poo.
- Rectal pressure so great you fear your anus may explode.
- More energy than the Duracell bunny.
- Your vulva feeling like it's being stretched out like a marquee as baby crowns.
- A slippery sensation as baby slops out of your snatch like a wet otter.

But what will pushing a tiny human out of your snatch actually feel like? Well, having a baby descend through your vaginal passage feels much the same as the discomfort of having built up a gigantic shitty backlog in your bum passage and then attempting to release it. It's like the worst constipation you've ever had, but imagine that the turd you're trying to expel is made of concrete, weighs 8lb and is travelling completely unlubed through your internal organs. The pressure of such a large, seemingly unmalleable object travelling down through your insides will of course be felt in your pelvis, but it can also feel pronounced in your fanny and in your bumhole – quite literally. What with the bearing down and the extra blood pumping round your lower half, your undercarriage is now likely to be resembling the swollen genitalia of a horny baboon on heat. You're essentially the owner of two puffed-up Mick Jagger vag lips and a bulbous cauliflower bumhole. Birth is just so fucking beautiful.

For the birthing partner

For the mum, auntie, partner, best mate – whoever gets the privilege of being present for the birth – here are some tips to help get your labouring loved one (and you) through the experience.

Be prepared. The best thing to prepare both you and your preggo partner for birth is research. Read the birthing books, go to the antenatal classes, familiarise yourself with the breathing techniques, understand the medical jargon around birth, talk to your partner about what she wants and basically arm yourself with the knowledge needed to bust your way into that delivery room knowing exactly what she needs to feel supported.

Take control. Once labour has started, it's your job to act as your partner's PA (Punani Assistant). You should deal with all the birth admin from timing contractions, getting the bags ready if you're going to hospital, making sure your partner has everything she needs, making sure the environment is just right, fielding queries from midwives, asking questions if you need to, being her advocate if she's unhappy about a procedure. It's your job to be her voice so that she can focus solely on birthing the baby.

Be engaged. Put your phone away, roll up your sleeves and get ready to get your hands dirty ... or at least ready to manhandle the odd stray turd. Offer her a back rub, fetch her a drink, try to second-guess her every need so she doesn't have to ask. Hold her hand, dab her forehead with a cold damp cloth, help her get into the most comfortable position, guide her through her breathing and keep telling her what an incredible job she's doing and to keep going even when she screams 'this is all your fault you fucking wanker'. She doesn't mean it. Well, she sort of does but throughout this labour she's going to need you.

Stay calm and positive. As important as it is for your partner to stay calm during the labour, it's equally beneficial for you. Not only will it help to keep you focused on the job of looking after her as best you can, but your serenity will also rub off on her, resulting in one massive oxytocin-jizzing love orgy. There may come a moment when she starts to doubt herself or labour starts moving in an unprecedented, potentially scary direction when you need to be her reassurance that everything is going to be OK and make her feel as safe as possible – even when you're literally shitting a brick in your undercrackers.

Scoop the poop. Mate, just take one for the team and dispose of that hot doodoo without her ever noticing. If she doesn't realise it's happened, she never needs to know. Take it to the grave, baby!

Push it real good

Up until this point, the focus has been on staying calm and chill to keep that vag-friendly love juice, oxytocin, flowing freely so your labour can progress with ease. Unlike during the first stage of labour, where stress hormones such as adrenaline and cortisol would have slowed down or even halted birth, your body will now actively release these bad boys to help create powerful, effective contractions that push baby down your vaginal canal. This switch-up is all part of the physiological wonder of birth and functions to literally eject your baby from your womb as quickly and safely as possible.

   As a result of this rise in adrenaline, the hazy stoner trance you may have found yourself in during the earlier stage of labour is now replaced with an altogether more alert and vivacious pizazz. I like to refer to this stage as the awakening of your inner warrior woman. With each contraction the laid-back, loved-up, pan-pipe-toting hippy that you channelled in stage one dissipates to reveal one bad-ass feisty bitch, poised and ready to conquer. SHE IS FIERCE and this mighty rush of energy should hopefully put the wind right back in your flaps to get you through this challenging stage of labour.

Once the urge to push has kicked in, it will ebb and flow in conjunction with your contractions. The midwives are likely to advise when you should and shouldn't be pushing, but in my experience, once your body has started the process (which it does involuntarily), there's not much you can do to stop it. The key, really, is to listen to your body and try to work in synchronisation with whatever it's doing to make sure each push is as powerful and intentional as possible. No dicking about, guys, make every push count and this shit will be over before you can say 'can I have a new vagina please?'

How the hell do I do that then, mate? Well, you should be familiar with the sensation of a contraction building by now, so as soon as you feel it rising, take a few deep breaths and get ready to squeeze. When you reach the peak of your contraction, use the momentum that your body has naturally created to bear down, just like when you strain for a poo, with as much vigour as you can muster.

Now as a warning, with all this pushing you may inadvertently curl a turd or two off without even realising you're doing it. Again, don't be scared by the prospect of this happening; it's incredibly common and nothing to feel embarrassed or ashamed about. Remember what I told you before, the midwives have seen it all, babes, so a cheeky bum nugget slipping out of your arsehole is not going to faze them. Plus, there's nothing funnier than watching your partner fish your shit out with a miniature net from the birthing pool.

Once you've pushed the baby far enough down your love tunnel, it will reach its final hurdle – your flaps – and the process of crowning will begin. You'll be aware this is underway when a new sensation is thrown into the general mix of 'what the fuck is happening?' pain radiating from your foof, as the baby's head pushes against your vulva. You may start to feel a tingling, stinging or burning sensation that grows steadily stronger as your peachy pocket stretches out to unimaginable proportions to accommodate your baby's emerging skull.

At the point of crowning (when your baby's head exits your vagina) the feeling will intensify as your beef curtains reach their maximum elasticity. This is often referred to as 'the ring of fire' as it literally feels like your vagina is being subjected to a continuous friction burn. As Johnny Cash sang, it burns, burns, burns. But the moment is fleeting and at any second, your baby's head will cross the threshold of your fanny and penetrate your labia with a pop. Oh, the relief!

The hard part is over but you're not quite done yet. It'll feel a tad weird for a few moments as the baby's head just casually dangles between your legs, but a few more pushes and, hey presto, your baby will be gliding out of your battered hole like a well-greased cannonball. You smashed it, mate! The sprog is out, your vagina is in pieces but the shitshow is almost over and, most importantly, you finally get to hold your baby in your arms. All those months spent waiting for this moment and here it is. You're a mum. Welcome to motherhood, bitches!

Intervention

As I've reminded you consistently, pregnancy and labour can take a number of unexpected twists and turns and sometimes intervention is necessary. If at any point the medical staff deem there is a danger to you or your baby, they will act accordingly. It's important to remember your birthing rights and to question the reasoning behind the medical professionals' decisions to intervene in your labour – ultimately it is your birth and they have to respect your autonomy over your body. Obviously, I'm not suggesting you refuse life-saving treatment, but as I've said before, do your research. Again, the AIMS website (www.aims.org.uk) contains up-to-date research on every aspect of childbirth plus information on your birthing rights within the UK, so read it!

As a brief overview, the most common interventions practised in the UK are:

Forceps and ventouse

If for any reason your baby experiences difficulty moving down your vaginal canal during the pushing phase or needs to be removed quickly due to safety concerns, forceps or a ventouse can be used to get baby out. You will be given an anaesthetic in your vagina and perineum before they are inserted, so you shouldn't feel too much. Sometimes an episiotomy (see below) is also needed to make the vaginal entrance bigger – as if we needed any more help with that.

Forceps

Ever played that arcade game where you have to control a giant metal claw to try to grab a prize out of a box? Well, that's essentially what forceps do – only the prize is a greased-up newborn and the box is your broken vag. Like a pair of large tweezers, they are inserted into your vagina, placed round the baby's head and then used to guide baby out of your hole. Sometimes forceps can leave small contact marks or bruises on your baby's face.

Ventouse

Ever had a massive turd block your drain and had to suction out the obstruction with a plunger? Yeah, well essentially, that's exactly what a ventouse does – it's a pum-pum plunger. The ventouse cup is literally suctioned on top of baby's head and then guided down your vag canal. As you can imagine, it's not the most comfortable procedure, but it's possibly less intrusive than forceps. Again, ventouse can leave small marks or bruises on baby's skull and can sometimes give baby the appearance of a tropical fruit – like an elongated banana head. But don't worry, this will soon return to normal.

Episiotomy

An episiotomy is an incision made in the perineum during labour if baby needs to be delivered quickly. Yep, there's no polite way of putting it – you're going to be sliced a new bumhole. Eeeeek! The cut is administered to make the entrance to your vagina wider so baby can be swiftly removed. You will be given an anaesthetic locally or if you've had an epidural you probably won't feel a thing. You most likely will need stitches after labour and sitting down comfortably might not be an option for a while until the cut heals.

Emergency or unscheduled Caesarean section

If you need an emergency C-section, a doctor has decided that you or your baby are in dire stress and immediate delivery is the only option. An unscheduled C-section is slightly different in that it's still considered urgent, but typically mother and baby aren't in a life-threatening situation. These are normally performed when labour hasn't progressed, contractions are weak or baby isn't tolerating labour, as opposed to there being significant risk to either the mother or baby's life.

An emergency C-section can be performed in as little as a few minutes if necessary. If you had an epidural while you attempted vaginal delivery, there may be enough time to give you additional medicine through your epidural so you can be awake during the procedure. If you didn't have an epidural, then your doctor may have to give you a general anaesthetic (meaning you won't be awake during the event) and you'll meet your baby when you wake up.

Non-emergency C-sections, for example one being performed because labour hasn't progressed normally, usually begin within 30 to 60 minutes of your doctor making the decision. You'll probably get to be awake for this C-section and meet your baby immediately. You'll get a spinal anaesthetic, an epidural, or a combination of the two, so you won't feel any pain.

Emergency and unscheduled Caesareans carry different risks compared with elective Caesareans, but both procedures involve making an incision through the abdomen and uterus to deliver your baby. As you can imagine, recovery from a C-section is typically much longer than from a vaginal birth. A C-section wound will take around six weeks to heal, during which time it is advised that you rest as much as possible and avoid lifting anything other than your baby.

Stage 3: delivery of the placenta

But don't rest on your laurels just yet as there's still the small matter of expelling your placenta. Either your body will do this of its own accord or the midwife will administer an injection of oxytocin to speed up the process. This is called active management and is now recommended for all women. You can opt out of this but make sure it's discussed with your midwife before delivery and is included in your birth preferences. Either way, your placenta shouldn't be knocking about inside you for much longer than approximately an hour after giving birth.

When the baby is born, it will still be attached to the placenta via the umbilical cord, which will continue to pump blood into your baby's system for a few minutes after birth. Evidence suggests that it's better not to cut the umbilical cord immediately, due to this transfer still taking place, so ask the midwife to wait between one and five minutes before going in for the snip.

Once cut, you will have approximately 60cm of now-defunct umbilical cord dangling casually from your vag like a giant tampon string made of human gristle, but don't worry, it'll be making its way out of you soon. If you've been left to deliver your placenta without active management, once it's detached from your womb, you will feel your uterus contracting until it's expelled out of your vag with a slop. If you've had active management, the midwife may help the placenta out by using your umbilical tampon string to perform a controlled cord contraction. Either way, your fanny will probably resemble a well-burrowed warren after birthing a child so it should just tumble out of your minge with a bounce and you'll barely notice a thing.

At this point the placenta is checked over by the midwife to make sure it has exited your uterus in one piece and you may be asked whether you'd like to see it too. Great if you know what the hell you're looking at but personally, they could have shown me a pig's digestive tract and I'd have been none the wiser. If you want to retain the placenta for consumption (excuse me while I throw up in my mouth) or for placenta encapsulation (where you pay one million pounds to have it freeze-dried and put into capsules) make sure the midwives are aware of your intentions so it doesn't end up in the incinerator rather than the frying pan.

Immediately after birth

Once the drama of labour is finally over and your uterus has been well and truly emptied, you're probably wondering what the hell happens next. First and foremost, you and baby will be checked over by the midwife/doctor to make sure everything is hunky dory (although it'll be more hunky gory in the case of your fanny). You'll have your blood pressure, pulse and temperature checked and if you had a vaginal birth, your perineum and vaginal wall will also be checked for any tears that need repairing with stitches (see the next chapter for more on that). They'll also feel your tummy to make sure your womb is shrinking back to its normal size. In the case of a C-section, you will remain in theatre while your incision is stitched up.

While all this is going on, you'll be given plenty of opportunity to bond with your newborn, skin to skin, and may even attempt your first breastfeed (more on this in Chapter 10). You'll also be offered something to eat and will get to shower off the mucky debris of birth. Your partner should be able to stay with you the entire time during this process and even overnight if allowed. If you have a home birth, the midwife will stay with you for the initial checks and then come back later that day to check in on you and your baby.

During the first eight hours post birth, the midwife will need to see you pass urine. Don't worry, she won't be examining your battered beefcake with binoculars as you pee, but she'll want to check that your piss pipes are functioning as they should be after birth. Difficulty passing urine, or urinary retention, as it is known, is a common problem in the first day or two following childbirth. Not surprising really, given the trauma your puss has just suffered in getting your baby out. Causes of a reluctant urethra include soreness, vaginal swelling, having an epidural, damage from tearing/forceps/episiotomy.

Now as you can imagine, passing a hot stream of acidic liquid through your delicate hole is not exactly going to be pleasant. Bit like rubbing some salt on a papercut, only the papercut is one massive vaginal-shaped wound. To get your wee wee flowing freely and to help this eye-watering moment pass with minimum ouch, you can do the following:

- Neck water like a thirsty camel. It'll simultaneously keep you weeing frequently and dilute the acidity of your piss.
- Take painkillers to ease the discomfort of your bulbous undercarriage, which may help you relax.
- Get up and walk around. You don't need to reach your 10,000 daily steps, but just a little bit of movement may help you to pass urine.
- Get some privacy. No one likes an audience, but especially not when you feel your uterus may slip out of you at any given moment.
- Piss in the shower or bath. The warmth of the water will help you to relax and make it easier to dribble out your daisy.

If you are still unable to pass urine eight hours after the birth of your baby, your midwife or a doctor will need to empty your bladder using a urinary catheter. This is a thin, sterile tube, which is usually made of plastic and is passed into your urethra (the small opening through which urine is passed) and into your bladder. This allows the urine to drain out. Having a catheter inserted can be a little uncomfortable but it is a quick, safe procedure. It may be necessary to leave the catheter in place for 24–48 hours to let the bladder 'rest'. If this happens, a drainage bag will be attached to the catheter to collect the urine.

If you've given birth in hospital or a midwife unit and you and your baby are well, you'll probably be able to go home between 6 and 24 hours after your baby is born. If you've had a home birth, the midwife will probably leave a couple of hours after the birth and return within 24 hours to make sure you are both OK. If you have a C-section, you will be in hospital for at least two days after birth becoming going home. Ask your hospital/birthing centre what to expect for your length of stay.

Going home with your new baby in tow is when the real fun begins!

C-section

Hello C-sectioners. I hope you haven't been reading this chapter thinking, what a bitch, she hasn't once mentioned what happens when your dream of the perfect birth goes up in flames like a paper bag full of shit on a doorstep and you're rushed for emergency surgery to remove your baby. Ladies, I see you. I've witnessed first-hand from family and friends what you've been through and let me tell you – all I have is the utmost respect for what your body has been through and by no means have you been overlooked.

I've spoken to many women who have had emergency C-sections and I've seen the range of emotions that come with the experience. From feeling deep disappointment that their body had somehow failed them (it didn't), through to sadness and a sense of loss of not being able to birth their child 'naturally', then the shame they've been made to feel by other people simply because their child wasn't born out of their vagina. If you're one of those women or you're reading this and thinking, yeah but having a C-section isn't really giving birth, you need to stop right now because it's BULLSHIT. However you give birth – out of your minge, via surgery, out of your fucking nostrils (which would probably be easier, tbf), no one route is more valid. So don't be that idiot who thinks having a C-section is a walk in the park, because it's not!

Having a C-section is hardcore surgery that takes its toll both physically and mentally, from limited mobility post-surgery, to longer recovery times, to impacting on breastfeeding. That's a lot to take on board, yeah! So this is really a message for all the women out there who have either undergone, are planning a C-section, or end up having an emergency C-section during birth. I want you to repeat the following:

- You do not need to squeeze a baby out of your vagina for it to qualify as giving birth.
- Your worth as a woman is not defined by the method it took to get your baby out.
- You are not a failure.
- Anyone who ever comments negatively about how you birthed is a cunt.
- You are amazing and incredible and just be thankful that your minge is still in one piece.
- Becoming a parent is a journey and the path your baby takes coming into this world, whether out of your hole or your stomach, bears no relation to your ability to mother them.
- Fuck anyone else who thinks otherwise, you absolute legend. And on the bright side, at least you can still look at your vagina without being reminded of a Picasso painting.

You've got this

Now I realise that I've painted quite a picture of birth here, and my intention was never to scaremonger or make you feel afraid. Quite the opposite, in fact. I hope that by sharing this honest perspective on what it may feel like going through labour will help you feel somewhat prepared for the task ahead.

Personally, giving birth was up there with one of the most empowering experiences of my life and left me feeling I was capable of anything. Of course it hurt beyond comprehension, and of course there were moments when I felt unable to continue, but somehow I got through it and survived to tell the tale. And that's just it – however your birth plays out, whether it's easy and straightforward or riddled with complications, just know that everything you experience, no matter how painful or traumatic, is temporary and WILL end.

Women give birth every day, in a world in which we often set ourselves very high standards. It's easy to fall into the comparison trap and pitch our own experiences against those of others. Sure, some women will give birth without pain relief, calmly and serenely, at home or in birthing pools, while a pan pipe gently plays in the distance and she births harmoniously out of her chakra. But equally, there are thousands of women who scream like deranged banshees, neck every drug going and deliver their baby in a shower of their own faeces. Just because your birth doesn't look the same as that of some other bints, it doesn't mean you've been less brave or stoical or brilliant than you should have been.

Giving birth isn't a competition, babes, it's a heroic and extraordinary thing to do. You should feel proud of yourself for facing and experiencing this huge challenge, however many drugs you did or didn't take and whatever way your baby made its entrance. There's no such thing as the perfect labour, so expect nothing to go to plan, embrace whatever happens and know that at the end of this epic journey, the greatest reward will be waiting for you. Your baby.

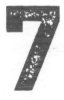

THE AFTERMATH

Don't look down

So you got the baby out. Well bloody done. You survived nine arduous months of being slowly sucked dry by a hungry foetus and triumphantly battled your way through a *Krypton Factor* of clunge challenges to give birth. You absolute legend! However it went, good or bad, all that hard work has finally paid off and here you are with your tiny bundle of joy safely in your arms. Your cervix may feel like it's been pummelled repeatedly by a small Transit van and your swollen flaps might be hanging forlornly like two beefy hammocks between your knees, but none of it matters – you're a mum!

Now that the baby has officially expelled itself from your uterus, you have entered the final stage of your pregnancy and birth experience; the fourth trimester. What the f is that?! I hear you cry. I thought I was done with those pesky trimesters. Well, almost. The fourth trimester refers to the twelve-week period immediately after you have had your baby and is a time of great physical and emotional change as your baby adjusts to being outside the womb, and you adjust to your new life as a mum.

This chapter will focus on the physical challenges you face during this period, with the emotional and mental impact of new parenthood saved for the next chapter. So now the baby is out, what's next for your body? Much like during your pregnancy, your postnatal bod is going to go through all sorts of unexpected physical and emotional adjustments as it begins to recover and heal after pregnancy and birth. You may begin to notice these changes pretty quickly and could find yourself questioning what the hell is happening to your body just hours after your baby has popped out of your foof. For example, you may be concerned that your vagina is now a gigantic bucket that's roomy enough to smuggle a family of four through customs. Or you could be wondering whether the chunks of uterus that look like roofing insulation falling out of your minge are normal. Or if it's OK that you're suddenly sweating out of your under-boobs like a menopausal woman in a sauna.

This chapter should hopefully prepare you for what's in store physically during the first few hours and subsequent weeks of postpartum and what you can do to help aid your recovery. From healing your tattered bits to surfing the biggest crimson wave of your life, through to squeezing your first poo out past your freshly laid postpartum haemorrhoids, I will take you through every grimace and ouch moment to get your body (and your growler) back to its former glory. It'll take a while to shake the feeling of having been run over by a bulldozer, but don't worry, your battered cave of a minge won't feel this way forever. The body has remarkable healing powers and after a few months recovering, you'll be doing the splits in no time.

Frankenminge

The majority of women (90 per cent) who give birth vaginally will experience some form of disturbance in the foofoo department, be it a graze, a tear or an episiotomy. Most tears occur internally in the vagina and into the perineum. Once you have given birth, you will be assessed by a midwife to gauge the extent of the damage and then given stitches if needed.

There are different degrees of tearing, ranging from a teeny labia chafe through to full-blown perineum annihilation. The most common are first- and second-degree tears. The minge massacre scale is as follows:

First-degree tear. You've either been blessed with elasticated flaps or your baby has a head the size of a peanut because your minge has survived with minimum breakage. Normally only affecting the skin, your wounds will usually heal quickly and without treatment.

Second-degree tear. Remember how we laughed at perineal massage and said, 'not for me thanks, I'll be fine', well, guess who's having the last laugh now? Not your vagina, that's for sure – although ironically it does look like she's smiling now she extends 2cm into your perineum. This tear requires stitches and a few weeks of recovery.

Third-degree tear. Your baby has really done one over on you, the massive-headed wanker. The term 'ripped me a new arsehole' has never felt more apt. Extending through the perineum and into the muscle surrounding the anus, this tear often requires surgery and may take a bit longer than a few weeks to heal.

Fourth-degree tear. Involving your perineum, anal sphincter and the mucus membrane that lines the rectum, this is the mother of all tears. Who knows where it starts and where it ends. Like third-degree tears, this tear requires surgery and a longer recovery time.

Fixing up your pummelled pouch will involve anaesthetic, stitches and a high probability of expletives exiting your mouth. You will be asked to lie down with your legs raised in stirrups and a spotlight shone on your beaver so the midwife or healthcare provider can get to work. If you've had an epidural you shouldn't feel a thing, but if not, the areas requiring stitches will be injected with a local anaesthetic first, then sewn up neatly with a surgical needle and thread.

This was by far my least-favourite moment from both my birth experiences, and one I do not wish to repeat. For that reason, if you're offered gas and air for the pain (which it's likely you will be) don't be a numb-nut like me and say no. You'll need it. Thankfully, despite repeatedly shouting, 'stop, you bunch of fucking cunts' to the staff present at the procedure, they ignored me and finished the job successfully. Not my finest moment, but thanks to my midwife Modupe, I found the perfect epitaph for my tombstone – 'Victoria, I have never heard such dirty words come out of such a pretty mouth.' Silver linings and all that.

Once you've been trussed up like a Christmas gammon, you will be offered a suppository of pain relief which will be popped expertly up your newly sewn anus. I paint a grim picture here, and while – like everything in this crazy birth experience – it may make you want to rip your vagina off, just remember that it won't last forever.

As you can imagine, your entire downstairs department is going to feel really sore for the next few days. You may even question where your fanny starts and your bumhole ends as it just feels like you have one singular amalgamation of vagina and anus – a vaganus, if you like. It's going to be swollen and possibly bruised, so expect your lips to sit like a pufferfish on steroids in your undercrackers. This makes sitting down, moving and generally existing a tad uncomfortable, so rule out doing any star jumps for the foreseeable future. Your stitches should dissolve after two weeks, and you should heal within three to four weeks of your baby's birth. After two months you should be pain-free. See the healing tips on page 145 for some advice on what you can do to ease the transition from trussed-up Frankenminge to a semblance of normality. It'll take a few weeks of careful movements and walking like you've shat yourself, but in the meantime, there's plenty you can do to soften the discomfort, as shared later in this chapter. And rest assured, it will heal!

Carrie clunge

But don't relax just yet as there's still more to come for your beaten little bun in the form of your postpartum bleed. Similar to a period, this delightful womb gravy (known as lochia) is made up of leftover blood, mucus and uterine tissue and will discharge out of your hole for three to ten days after giving birth. As you've been cultivating this uterus batter to grow your baby for nine months, the flow of your bleed may be significantly heavier than your normal periods. You could in fact lose a whopping 500ml of blood before it begins to taper off, so don't be alarmed if your vagina ends up resembling Carrie on her prom night.

The consistency may also be different from your normal period, and the blood could have a thicker, gooier texture, with the odd clot or lump peppered amid the general gore. If you've been sitting or lying down for any length of time, the bleeding may pool and then gush when you stand or move – much like my experience of going to the loo first thing in the morning and my clam dramatically spraying a night's worth of pooled gunk across the bathroom like Spiderman shooting his web. An excellent party trick, I'm sure you'll agree, but not such a good look for your interiors. Unless, of course, you're going for the 'explosion at the tomato ketchup factory' vibe and enjoy crimson accents of minge sauce up your walls.

To manage your bleed, make sure you've stocked up with plenty of maternity specific pads or disposable pants. Wearing one feels like you've got an IKEA mattress wedged between your thighs, but unlike standard sanitaryware, they're designed specifically for the job of soaking up the excess of your womb entrails. Just make sure you change it frequently; it'll become sodden in no time, which is why a normal sanitary towel isn't fit for purpose. And forget about using tampons – not that I imagine you're harbouring a burning desire to shove a cotton bullet up your broken foof right now, but avoid the fanny plugs entirely for this bleed. Not only can they create infections but you may inadvertently cause even more damage to your already traumatised twat.

It's also worth picking up some disposable puppy training pads. Excuse me? Am I a fucking Labrador?! Trust me, they are the postpartum fanny's best friend. You aren't expected to take a piss on it but sleeping on one for the first few nights will protect your mattress against any leaks. Plus, if you want to air your clunge out for a bit, you can get your flaps out on the sofa without worrying about ruining your upholstery.

As mentioned, the initial heavy bleed may last anywhere from three to ten days before easing off and returning to a daily discharge. This may be red at first but will gradually turn to a watery pink, then brown and finally to a yellowish white. Just remember that the flow is different for everyone and if you have any concerns or believe your bleeding is excessive, contact your medical healthcare provider immediately.

Contractions

I bet you've read the title to this section and exclaimed, 'Contractions?! Are you fucking kidding me! I thought that shit was over!' Well, I'm sorry to inform you that the quimquakes don't end immediately with delivery. As it stands, your uterus is currently flapping about inside you like a carrier bag on a windy day, so your body is going to need to do some work to get it back to its pre-pregnancy size and position. Your uterus will continue to contract for the first few days to a couple of weeks after birth, and with each contraction it will shrink down, descend back into your pelvis and help to slow the tsunami of lochia pum-pum plasma currently flowing out of your flange.

Unlike labour contractions, there is no pattern to when or how often these afterpains will strike and they do not grow in intensity or last for a sustained period of time. No beating around the battered bush here, they hurt, but how strongly you feel them will be down to your individual threshold of pain and whether you've had previous pregnancies or have experienced excessive stretching (as with a multiple pregnancy). The bigger your bin bag of a uterus, the more uncomfortable it's going to be reining it in.

Afterpains can also be more intense during breast-feeding. This is due to the oxytocin that is released in the process of letting down your milk, which as we know from birth, is the integral hormone for driving uterine contractions. I can testify to this as my uterus always perked up when a baby was sucking on my tit. Ironically, despite the love drug spurting out of my brain, those first few weeks of feeding felt like I had baby piranha attached to my areola, so not only did I have the sensation of my nipples being gnawed off to deal with, I then had the added joy of my womb convulsing like it was being kicked repeatedly by a pair of steel-capped Dr Martens. Fantastic! There is some relief, though, as you can manage the pain with paracetamol and ibuprofen (see the healing tips in this chapter). I found using my Barry sex-pest breath from labour was also beneficial and would huskily exhale like a sex offender through most breastfeeds.

Luckily this whole process of uterine shrinkage is relatively quick and any afterpains should subside naturally within four to seven days. By the end of your first week post-birth, your bucket of a womb will have already reduced by half, and if your healing is on track, by your sixth week it should be back to its normal size.

Poo gate

At some point in these first few hazy, crazy, vaginally harrowed days of motherhood, you need to be mentally and physically prepared for the fourth and final stage of labour – your first poo. I know what you're thinking, how the hell can you shit comfortably when it feels like one misjudged strain and your puffed-up patchwork tapestry of a perineum will explode all over the toilet pan? Not to mention getting said turd past the fistful of post-partum dangleberries currently hanging out of your bum. How is it possible to shit without your insides falling out?

Now I'm not going to lie, it's going to be anal Armageddon, but unless you want to end up in A&E having compacted faeces surgically removed from your back passage, you need to poo. However, all is not lost at sphincter sea and there are a few little bumhole-friendly steps you can follow to help prepare your vaganus for the inevitable passing of your first stool.

First and foremost, don't hold it in! The longer you leave it, the bigger and harder that turd will grow, and before you know it, it'll feel like you're trying to shit a breeze block through a Cheerio. Feel the urge – brace for impact.

Stool softeners are your friend. Remember the powdered magnesium citrate from your constipated pregnancy days? Get on it. Start necking that poo-softening magic asap and make sure you're eating a healthy balanced diet that includes your five portions of fruit and veg a day – jeez, I'd go so far as to snort a line of Brussels sprouts if it eased the descent of that dump.

Release the fear and the turds will flow. We're all familiar with hypnobirthing now and the same concept applies to shitting, just try to relax and breathe! Get your anal zen on and visualise your battyhole opening up like a beautiful (if slightly deformed) rosebud.

Use a warm, damp flannel to apply gentle counter pressure to your broken Betsy. It should ease the sensation of your uterus/anus falling out and as an added bonus, you can leave the flannel out for your partner's daily facial wipe down. I mean, they are partly responsible for this situation so why not get a bit of payback?

Use your Gollum squatty potty from pregnancy and ensure your feet are raised – in fact, this should become a permanent fixture in your daily shitting regime. There are so many benefits to using a squatty potty to take a poo, especially when you have the fear of vaganus eruption kicking off. Not only will it reduce the amount you need to strain (due to the alignment of your intestines with your feet raised) but it will also encourage pelvic floor engagement as you curl one off. Easy shitting and a tighter vag – win, win.

Bertie the bum grape

On the subject of your anus, I think it's time to address the elephant in the room – or rather, the elephant hanging out of your bumhole. Vaginal labour can be a bit of a bitch to your botty and wreak havoc on your ring. The pushing and straining that comes with birthing a baby creates internal pressure in your back passage and can literally force blood vessels in your anal passage to swell and subsequently pop out of your bumhole. So you may find that in addition to welcoming your bundle of joy, your bottom may also welcome its own bundle of fleshy postnatal haemorrhoids. As we discussed earlier, some of you will have already been blessed with these anal appendages during pregnancy, and if so, labour will have almost definitely aggravated the pesky drupes, further augmenting your swollen anus.

However they got there, either in pregnancy or during labour, be warned – the aftermath of anal annihilation can rival the pain of your pounded pum-pum. For some, this extra botty sinew won't be a bother at all, but for others it'll feel like you're walking around with a kilo of raw ulcerated bum meat hanging out of your arse.

I was one such victim of this heinous haemorrhoid suffering. The damage to my derriere was so excruciating that, at moments, I genuinely believed my bottom was going to implode. I knew the birth had hit me hard in the anal department, as I spent the majority of the pushing stage fearing that I was going to shit out my lower intestines or that my sphincter would burst. This fear was confirmed by my mum announcing shortly after birth that she had glanced down between my legs to see what was going on and was greeted by the sight of, her words, 'a gigantic fucking cauliflower' protruding from my bum. The aftermath was intense. I'd had piles throughout pregnancy but these were like nothing I'd experienced before. They were hot and raw and furious, plus they were huge! It felt like I was smuggling a grapefruit in my pants, so sitting down was near impossible and trying to squeeze a poo out felt like I was shitting glass.

About three days after giving birth, the pain was so intense that it woke me up. I lay in the darkness silently crying, as my anus throbbed rhythmically with blood pulsating through its gnarly girth. 'Wait a minute,' I thought, 'the pulsations – they're like Morse code. Maybe it's trying to communicate with me!' But what was it trying to tell me? The meaning of life? The answer to happiness? Or was it just saying, 'GO TO THE DOCTOR YOU FUCKING IDIOT, THIS ISN'T NORMAL'. I took its advice and the next morning booked an emergency appointment to have my cavity assessed by a medical professional.

As fate would have it I was sent to a surgery miles away from my house and to a doctor I had never seen before. Having left Rob and baby at home (she was combi-feeding so I wasn't worried about needing to breastfeed) I made the hairy taxi ride alone. Trying not to scream from the impact of every speed bump on my bumhole, I was dropped off at the wrong location and had to walk for an agonising ten minutes, fighting back the tears. Every step chafed my bum boulder into an even angrier rage and I arrived at the clinic flustered, sweating profusely and on the verge of a breakdown. Withing minutes, I was called to the consultation room. As I delicately pigeon-stepped towards the door, it suddenly occurred to me that I was potentially going to have to bare my broken bumhole to this unknown doctor and I immediately started praying, 'please be a female, please be a female, please be a female'. Lo and behold, I opened the door and who should be sitting at the desk but a MAN! Of course it was a man and of course he was good-looking. Well, this trip can't get any worse, I thought, but indeed it could.

After an in-depth conversation about the state of my slaughtered sphincter, Dr Good-looking turned to me and said, 'Would you just like to pop yourself up on the bed over there and we'll take a look at what we're dealing with.' Oh Lord. I reluctantly agreed. 'I'll just close the curtain so you can have some privacy and then I'll come in, OK?' Meanwhile, I'm thinking – Love, you're about to inspect my arsehole, I really don't think the curtain staying open is going to be an invasion of my privacy right now. So there I am, minge, arsehole, the whole mess just laid out, raw and ready for analysis. He comes back in and instructs me to face the wall and raise my knees towards my chest. I do as I'm told and as I lay there in the foetal position, staring at the paint cracking on the wall and wondering what the hell had happened to my life to end up here with my bottom laid out on a table like a bumhole buffet, I hear the distinct snap of a pair of latex gloves being pulled on. Oh here we go, I thought. 'I'm just going to have a little feel now, Mrs Emes,' he says, pulling my cheeks tentatively apart. A little feel, OK, I can deal with a little feel – next thing I know he's gone straight in for my giblets, no warm-up, no warning, just a sharp poke with his lubed-up index finger followed by a thorough foraging around the perimeter of my arsehole. 'Yes, I can see the problem here,' he said. See it? Mate, you're knuckle deep in the fucking problem, at the very least I hope you can see it! At this point I didn't know whether to laugh or cry at the absolute absurdity of me curled up getting my ruined anus fingered by a handsome stranger while praying to god that all the prodding didn't accidentally release a fart or, worse, a turd.

Thankfully my anus withstood the pressure of his digits and the whole humiliating encounter swiftly came to an end. A prescription for industrial suppositories and starfish numbing gel was issued and I shuffled out of that surgery hoping I'd never have to look that doctor in the eye, or the anus, ever again.

So what do you do with a ripe cluster of angrily throbbing bum nuggets hanging out of your back passage? How do you treat this postnatal anus ache? Of course you can seek medical assistance if needed, but there's a lot you can do at home. If you remember from the birth chapter, I shared several bulbous botty easing tips, so go back to page 29 for a quick refresher in anal care. And for further advice, you can also refer to the undercarriage healing guide on page 145.

You'll be pleased to know that haemorrhoids do shrink of their own accord and you'll be amazed at how rapidly they can deflate and disappear. Incredibly, despite having resembled a genetically modified cauliflower, my sphincter returned to its neatly puckered former self about two months after giving birth and I could once again fart without fear of shitting out my insides. However, for most people (including me) the bumgrapes never truly leave you, they just temporarily retreat back up your anus and occasionally pop out to say hello. This can be due to constipation, excessive straining and overexertion, so stay hydrated, use all your poop tools from the recovery guide and never, ever, stop taking your magnesium citrate supplements.

Healing tips

Having twice nursed a traumatised postpartum minge while dealing with the world's largest postnatal haemorrhoids, here are some tips and tricks I've picked up along the way to aid the healing process of your undercarriage. The aim here is to manage your pain, reduce swelling and bruising and reactivate that loose hammock of a pelvic floor muscle after birth.

The important thing to remember is that however rotten you feel physically in the first few days, time is the best and biggest healer. It'll take a couple of weeks before you can piss without feeling like your uterus is going to slide out of your cavernous bucket of a vag, but have faith, you'll get there.

Aquafresh pum

Plain lukewarm water is the post-partum fanny's BFF (battered flaps friend) and can be used in a variety of ways to bring your lady garden some light relief. Obviously cleanliness is paramount in your recovery, so keep your foof and surrounding areas as fresh as possible by washing regularly, changing your sanitary towel frequently and keeping perfumed soaps or creams at bay.

A few simple ways you can use water to provide pain relief:

- Submerge your snatch in a lukewarm bath – it's relaxing and takes the edge off the sting. Keep it brief – ten minutes is enough and won't compromise your stitches.
- For a cooling fanny spray, fill a spritz bottle with plain water and whack it in the fridge. When your hoof is feeling hot and bothered, a quick spray of this should bring immediate chilly relief.
- Invest in an elastic gel ice pack. This frozen fanny aid can be wrapped in a tea towel and shoved into your knickers, bringing relief as well as helping to reduce swelling. Also excellent for your bum grapes. If you don't have an ice pack, soak a sanitary towel in water (you can also add witch hazel) and pop in the freezer to create your own.
- Use a piss jug for urinating (see next paragraph).

Get your jugs out for the lads

So we've gone into quite some detail about preparing for your first dump post labour, but what about going for a wee?! Obviously we wee a hell of a lot more frequently than we shit and getting piss past your stitched-up perineum is going to sting. This is where the humble water jug is elevated to superhero status. That's right, keep a small jug next to the bog and every time you need to tinkle, fill it up with lukewarm water and pour it over your vag as you wee. It'll feel like magic fairy juice is cascading over your knackered flaps – well, not quite, but it simultaneously dilutes the acidity of your pee so reduces the burn and keeps your fanny squeaky clean in the process. Remember to gently dab once you're done, as opposed to wiping, to minimise any damage to stitches.

Airing your fairy

Ever been confined in a windowless room and the central heating whacked up full blast? It's suffocating! And that's exactly how your fanny is going to feel being under wraps 24/7. Airing out your bits for as little as ten minutes daily provides a much-needed break from the sweaty confines of a sanitary towel and gives your car crash of a clam the chance to breathe. Personally, I liked to save this moment for the evening, when my husband and I settled down for our nightly dose of Netflix. I would lay out a puppy toilet training pad on the sofa, whack my bottoms off and sit, spread-eagled, with my kebab blowing in the breeze while we delved into a documentary about serial killers – which seemed apt given that my nunny resembled the aftermath of a gruesome murder scene.

Painkillers

For the first few days after birth, it's highly likely that you're going to hurt, and not just in the genital region. Doesn't matter how the baby got out, giving birth can be physically brutal and you may feel like every inch of you has been put through a mangle. You're going to need a lot of rest, so chill your beans and lie down, do nothing and sleep at every given opportunity. If you need some help getting through the aches and pains you can take paracetamol and ibuprofen. These can be taken at the same time or spaced apart to provide 24-hour relief. Follow the instructions on the label or leaflet about how to take the medicines, and make sure you do not take too much of either. It's not recommended to take painkillers consistently for longer than three days, though, so consult your GP if you feel you still need to.

Alongside these, you can also take the homeopathic herbal remedy, arnica. This popular postpartum healer is believed to reduce bruising and stimulate muscle repair as well as provide pain relief, so it's the perfect antidote for your aching, fatigued faja jay. Take this orally for maximum benefit.

Loosey goosey

Not that you'll want to, but now is not the time for dressing in anything remotely labia skimming, like skinny jeans or Lycra. Keep your pantaloons and drawers loose with ample gusset room for maximum flap-swinging space and wear breathable materials like cotton or linen to keep your fairy nice and airy.

Pelvic floor exercises

I'm hoping you took my advice in Chapter 3 and worked on your pelvic floor muscles during your pregnancy. If so, well done and go strong, minge! All that 'vag-ercise' is going to stand you in good stead for your postnatal recovery, getting your vagina back in shape and preventing urinary incontinence. If you didn't get round to sculpting your VABs, don't worry, you can start now!

I know what you're thinking ... Are you mental? How the hell am I supposed to engage my minge muscles when it feels like they're made of jelly and my vaginal canal is just one big, cavernous hole? I hear you, sister, but the sooner you start trying to engage your pelvic floor after birth, the quicker your massive snatch will feel less like a suitcase. You should be familiar with the exercises by now (Ryan Gosling is eating your pussy and you don't want to fart on his face, remember) so get clenching as soon as you feel able. The first couple of attempts will no doubt feel futile, given that your entire vaginal canal has been stretched to Betsy, but persevere and you'll be flexing that fanny hammock like Schwarzenegger flexes his biceps in no time. Regular clenching should become a part of your daily routine, but it's easy to forget to do the exercises in the haze of looking after a newborn. It can be helpful to associate pelvic floor exercises with another daily activity you know you'll do without fail, like brushing your teeth or brushing your hair. Squeeze and brush, squeeze and brush!

Also see Chapter 12 for details on how to maintain long-term pelvic floor health.

It's getting hot in here

So as well as dealing with the wreckage that is your vagina, your flaps spurting blood, your uterus still randomly contracting and your anus presenting like a baboon on heat, you've got one last postnatal delight to deal with. The postpartum sweats!

Oh yes, things are about to get pretty hot and sweaty under the collar and, well, everywhere else too. Over the first few weeks post birth, you may find that your normally arid armpits are transformed into two liquid pools of sweat and you experience excessive perspiration that isn't just confined to your pits. Palms, feet, forehead, back of the knees, minge, underboobs – parts of you that have never released a bead of sweat until now will be spurting floods of bodily fluid.

But don't worry if you're suddenly sporting permanent damp patches; this is all perfectly normal and your clammy bits serve a very useful purpose. First, sweating rids your body of excess fluid, and boy did pregnancy bestow you with litres of that! Pregnancy increases your blood volume by an impressive 40 per cent, and once the baby is out, that extra blood needs to be reabsorbed by your body and excreted through urine and sweat. The second cause for that river of moisture flowing out of your underboob is the rapid decrease in oestrogen pumping through your body with the expulsion of your placenta. Oestrogen and progesterone levels are the highest in your life right before you deliver, but once the placenta is out, hormone levels rapidly drop, causing hot flushes and postpartum night sweats. The postpartum hormone drop is considered the single largest sudden hormone change in the shortest amount of time experienced by any human being, at any point of their life cycle. By about three days postpartum you're essentially back to a baseline that is close to non-pregnant. This stark hormonal drop also plays havoc with your emotions – think of the worst PMS you've ever had and then magnify it by 1,000. JOY! But we will come to that in greater detail in the next chapter.

Unfortunately, there's not much you can do to speed up this soggy process and some women will continue to sweat like a beast for several weeks or more, especially if breastfeeding. You're essentially experiencing what it feels like to be a menopausal woman – something else we have to look forward to in the future! Being a woman is fantastic ... You've just got to sweat this one out, ladies – literally! So keep necking the water to stay hydrated, invest in a decent deodorant and let your juices flow freely. If you experience hot flushes and sweat more at night, wear the bare minimum to bed and lay a towel down to sleep on so you don't end up in a pool of your own saline juices. And make sure the window is open to keep a breeze flowing around your burning flaps or, better still, aim a fan directly on to your body for maximum cooling comfort. Just try not to get downwind of your fanny on a hot night, else the dog will think you've brought pork chops home for dinner.

The good news is that all that additional finger/ankle/labia puff you gained over the last nine months will soon be exiting via your sweat glands and your piss hole and these parts will hopefully return to their pre-pregnancy bloat dimensions. So hooray for non-chipolata fingers!

Will I ever feel normal again?

Hopefully, having read this chapter you won't feel totally as freaked out when your body starts acting in mysterious ways post birth. We can focus so intensely on the labour part of childbirth that the postpartum period is often completely overlooked. This does us no favours, because the aftermath of giving birth can be just as brutal as the act itself. I wish I had been more prepared for just how difficult the first few weeks postpartum were going to be, because maybe then it wouldn't have hit me like such a massive bag of dicks. For some of us, it's going to be shitty, but I want you to know that however rough it gets, however broken your vagina may feel, one day the fog will lift and you'll be able to insert a tampon again without it involuntarily falling out.

The best thing you can do for yourself after having your baby is to show your body the love and kindness it deserves. What it has achieved through nurturing a foetus for nine months and the stress it went through being almost torn in half getting that sproglet out is nothing short of spectacular. As much as you feel like you want to 'bounce back' or go back to your pre-pregnancy self immediately, save it. That will come. These first few weeks should be about respecting the remarkable journey your body has been on and focusing on repairing and healing yourself from the inside out. So rest up my friend, cuddle your baby, eat good food, watch shit TV, get your partner to apply an ice pack to your haemorrhoids and get a nap in when you can. This is the time to heal. The rest is yet to come!

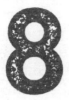

BIRTH STORIES

Now I couldn't talk about giving birth without sharing my own incredible labour experiences, so buckle up for a mingetastic tale of epic vag action.

As you know, I've had two children. Both were planned home births and both ended up exiting via my foof. I was pretty set on a home birth from the get-go, having been massively influenced by one of my best friends. Her experience of birth seemed so far removed from the horror stories I'd heard previously – she made it sound like giving birth was awesome and empowering. Listening to her, I didn't need much convincing, especially when I looked at the stats for intervention at home versus the hospital. Plus, I've always copied everything she's done because she's super cool and brilliant.

My births couldn't have been more opposite in terms of how they unfolded. Both had similar elements but how each stage progressed was completely different. That came as a big surprise to me, as I naively assumed they would be pretty much the same. But that's the wonderful thing about birth, right? You never know what the hell is going to happen!

My antenatal care was also completely different; first time round I was supported by a designated home-birth team and had the same amazing midwife, Laura, from twenty weeks all the way through to the birth. Second time, the home-birth team had been disbanded and I was in the care of the community midwives. I had several different people looking after me, with two midwives I'd never met present at the birth. This may seem insignificant, but it comes into play later on, so stay with me ...

The first perineum penetrator: Oliver

Oliver arrived at thirty-eight weeks plus five. As I described in the previous chapters, I was one of the 15 per cent of women whose waters broke before going into labour. I woke up at 6a.m. feeling the urge to wee, tottered down the hallway to the toilet and whoosh, with no warning, a bucket load of amniotic fluid gushed out of my fanny. With no sign of contractions at this point, I was told by my midwife to stay at home, relax and crack on with all the oxytocin-stimulating techniques I'd learned through hypnobirthing. I knew that if labour didn't start within 24 hours, I'd be recommended an induction, so I did everything within my power to try to get things moving.

After a full day of anxiously waiting for a sign that baby was coming, followed by an emotional breakdown when it didn't, I went to bed, resigned to the fact that I probably wasn't going to get the home birth I wanted.

This was probably around 9p.m. (don't judge me, I love an early bedtime). As soon as the lights went out and my head hit the pillow, I had my first contraction. From the onset, they came in thick and fast, starting at about thirty minutes apart and ramping up to five minutes apart in the course of an hour and a half. That is quick, especially for a first labour, and not at all what I was expecting. I spent this time either bent over a birthing ball or sitting on the toilet as my bowels violently emptied themselves between each contraction. A remarkable amount of poo exited me.

During this time, my husband, Rob, called my mum and the midwife. Mum was the first to arrive and made her entrance by exclaiming, 'It's bloody pitch black in here, I can't see a thing!' in her broad Birmingham accent. Things really started to hot up and contractions were now almost constant, with little respite between each one. Rob hadn't even had a chance to set up the birthing pool, so he disappeared downstairs to silently have a breakdown while panic-inflating the pool and filling it with 450 litres of water.

Meanwhile, Mum and I were upstairs when I suddenly had the urge to push. With no midwives on site yet (we called late, not realising how far along I actually was), despite not being able to see her face because it was so dark, I could sense the worry emanating from her as she was trying to calculate the logistics of delivering a baby by herself. Luckily, the first midwife, Sarah, showed up, and Mum's blood pressure returned to normal.

On Sarah's arrival, I was on the bed, on all fours, completely starkers, with my starfish on full display.

Sarah walked in, introduced herself (hadn't met her before) and I replied, 'Hi, I'm Victoria and this is my anus.' She laughed and then asked to perform a vaginal examination. I agreed and as soon as her digits passed the threshold of my flaps, they set off an intense contraction. She then scurried out of the room and I heard her whispering on the phone to my other midwife, Laura, who had supported me throughout my pregnancy, 'She's fully dilated, I repeat, fully dilated!' All in all, from the first contraction to fully open bagel cervix had taken two and a half hours, tops.

I don't remember how we got downstairs but the next thing I knew, I was in the birthing pool and the pushing was well and truly underway. At this point Laura arrived, and as soon as I saw her lovely face I felt completely at ease and filled with absolute confidence that I could do this.

Now unlike dilation, this stage took FOREVER. The urge to push came regularly, with plenty of downtime between each contraction, but it felt like Oliver moved down my vaginal canal a millimetre at a time. Each push moved him a teeny bit further, but as the power of each contraction ebbed away, it was like he retreated back into the depths of my uterus. It was basically like pushing out a concrete shit. After four hours of pushing to no avail, it was clear he needed some help exiting.

Everything felt really surreal and hypersensitized during this stage. I was tanked up on oxytocin and was genuinely off my head in the nicest possible way – like a raver hitting their peak after two Es and ten cans of Red Bull, but the only watermelon I was twisting was making its way down my cervix. On the advice of Laura, I got out of the pool and walked up the stairs to stretch my legs and hopefully encourage Oliver to get moving.

Had a couple of contractions on the loo and then made it back downstairs and into the pool again. But the water was almost too calming and relaxing, I was genuinely falling asleep in between contractions, so I got back out again and used Rob to hang off in a semi-squat position. Poor bloke.

I should note that for the majority of all this, the midwife had been applying pressure to my perineum as I pushed, but I hardly noticed it at all. Either way, the anal berries were well and truly presenting at this point and as my mum lovingly relayed to me afterwards, she looked down at one point and thought I was crowning. Well, I was, anally at least. In her words, 'It looked like a fucking cauliflower was coming out.' Thanks, Mum.

Getting out of the pool woke me up, the contractions kicked up a gear and Oliver suddenly made bigger lurches down my tunnel. I activated the old raspberry lips and began to feel the burn of his head breeching my flaps. Oh lord, the burn! And then with one almighty push, his head popped out with a scream (from me), tearing me a new one and suddenly I had half a baby hanging out of my clunge. Another push and out he slid like a slimy little otter.

Oh that feeling! Being so thankful that the ordeal of birth is over, mixed with the excitement of finally getting to meet your baby. It's incredible. Both physically and emotionally I was exhausted, but once my baby was plonked into my arms I didn't care about anything else. It was me, him and Rob against the world. We huddled together on the dining room floor, surrounded by bloodied towels, and cried tears of unadulterated joy staring down at the little creature we had made nine months before when I'd drunkenly mounted Rob in the night for a fondle.

At this point, Laura suggested we managed the delivery of the placenta with drugs. Oliver had exploded out of me in a heavy flow of blood so she wanted to err on the side of caution and get it out of me sooner rather than later. I agreed with no hesitation. She could have offered me heroin and I'd have said yes. I didn't give a shit what happened now the baby was finally out. And I really just wanted to lie down.

As I had torn, Laura had to stitch me back up, so while I showered with the help of my mum, Rob and the midwives were busy tidying up downstairs. I got through the ordeal of the stitches with Mum holding my hand and Rob holding Oliver and after being checked over and given the OK, everyone left. After all the commotion, all the busyness and energy of giving birth, it was finally just us. Rob, me and our brand-new baby snuggled up in bed with a cup of tea and some toast. I felt pretty fucking awesome, to be fair. I felt invincible. I was in awe of my body and what it had achieved and couldn't believe that my baby was finally here. I think I was pretty high on oxytocin because everything felt awesome. But yeah, it didn't last long. Pretty soon I was tits deep in the absolute shitshow of the postpartum period and I was a wreck. Fun times!

Second round of anal annihilation: Edith

Edith was born one hour past her due date. After a frustrating fortnight of false labour, I woke up that morning and went downstairs to have breakfast. As I sat mulling over my Weetabix, I felt a gooey deposit exit my fanny, stood up and there was my bloody show staring back at me! More uterus mucus with your cereal, dear?

I was pretty certain this meant labour was going to kick in at some point that day, so I shipped Oliver off to my mum's and got Rob to stay home from work, just in case I needed him. At about 1.30p.m. nothing had happened, so I decided to have a nap. Again, as soon as I lay down to sleep, I had my first contraction. Unlike my first labour, it was really mild, no more than a cramping, then I waited anxiously for the next one, hoping it wasn't a false alarm. Half an hour later, another contraction came and then they started coming regularly every 30–40 minutes. This lasted for a good few hours.

Progress felt slow, especially compared to my labour with Oliver, so by about 5p.m. I was getting impatient and wanted to speed things up. I'd already been indulging all my hypnobirthing techniques, but I got to work walking around the house, up and down the stairs and into the garden. Every step seemed to slowly but surely build up to a contraction and pretty soon they were getting closer and closer together while also gaining momentum. We rang triage and a community midwife was sent over. Let's call her Jean.

We'd never met Jean before and from the moment she arrived, she put me on edge. I put this down to her bedside manner as opposed to her professional capabilities – basically, she made me feel like a cunt. She was quite brash and didn't exude much warmth, which felt like a massive contrast to my previous experience with midwives at my birth. I felt I was an annoyance to her, especially as I refused vaginal examinations and asked her to monitor the baby's heartbeat from the position I was in, rather than lying on my back, which was incredibly painful. It was all a bit weird having her in my space, and very quickly my contractions dropped from being five minutes apart to twelve minutes apart. I wanted her out of the house (which I whispered aggressively to Rob in the kitchen), and as I was still pretty chill at this point, she said she would come back later. THANK GOD.

She left and I had to work really hard to get my contractions back up to speed by walking 18,394,039 miles around my house. During this time, Rob had prepared the birthing pool so it was all ready for me, but I held off getting in until my contractions were consistently close together. This probably took us up to about 11p.m., when everything suddenly became very intense. My contractions were really close together, lasting a long time, and the pain was becoming difficult to manage. We rang Jean and she advised not getting into the pool until she was there.

She arrived and just as I was about to get in the water, I thought it would be a good idea to do a quick cheeky poo to save soiling myself in the birthing pool. Halfway up the stairs I was hit by my biggest contraction yet and was doubled over mooing like a farm animal hanging on to the staircase. It felt like it lasted an absolute age, but when it finally subsided, I staggered to the toilet where I immediately had another contraction. With that contraction came the overwhelming urge to be sick and I called for Rob to come and help me.

He rushed upstairs and helped me to flip over so I was on all fours, dry-retching violently, with my head in the toilet and him standing behind me. Well, that was it. My body just automatically started pushing, but with such force that I started shitting uncontrollably. This wasn't normal shitting, but a cascading fountain of liquid poo literally falling out of my bumhole with absolutely no anal control. Remember that spicy curry I'd had the night before? Yeah, that was a mistake. Rob, god bless him, started cupping my shit in his bare hands to siphon it off, over my head, into the toilet. So there we were, me retching like *The Exorcist* with a stream of vindaloo falling out of my arse and Rob braced behind me, catching the hot mess of my innards. It was carnage. At this point my massive haemorrhoids were fit to burst and Rob, taking a break from cradling my poo, decided to try to pop them back in as a gesture of goodwill. The sensation of a digit on my bum as my cervix was simultaneously ripped to shreds was too much and I shouted, 'Rob, stop fingering my anus.' Oh, it was intense.

Obviously, hearing this commotion, the midwife made her way upstairs to help and got to work, crouching down at my minge using the light on her mobile phone (you know I like it dark in the birth cave) to illuminate my gaping holes. Unlike her brother, who had carefully and thoughtfully taken his time coming out, Edith was a callous monster. She came out of me with such force and speed I felt she was going to shoot across the room out of my minge like a human cannonball. And the sensation. OH MY LORDY! It was honestly like my pelvis was splitting in half as she nosedived out of me.

After a really slow start, this all happened so quickly and felt like it went from zero to one hundred in the space of seconds. But, thank god, it didn't last long and she busted through my flaps in a swift seventeen minutes. My first words when she finally plopped out were 'Oh my fucking god, my bumhole.' Precious.

At this point, the second midwife, Mopude, arrived and walked into what looked like a crime scene. There was blood and poo everywhere – Rob, Jean and I were covered in it and it STANK. Jean had it on her forehead, the poor bitch, and my feet took such a battering, it looked like I was wearing a pair of poo shoes. So yeah, if you're worried about shitting yourself, don't. It happens so frequently and it's really no big deal. We were cleaned up in no time and you'd never have known what had happened – although cupping handfuls of my shit will haunt Rob forever.

As Edith exitied at such velocity, I tore with her too, and because neither of the midwives felt confident to give me stitches at home, we were picked up by an ambulance and taken to the birthing centre. I was a bit disappointed that we had to go in, but it was necessary to patch up my gaping minge. A few hours later we were discharged and back home with our baby girl.

So there you have it, a brief insight into my experiences of birth for proof that no two births are ever the same, even between your own children. I know I've said it before, but I fucking love birth. It's absolutely mental and, yes, it hurts like a bitch, but I'd do it all over again in a heartbeat. I just can't be arsed with the pregnancy bit or actually having another kid, but the labour bit, I'll take it.

Nothing has ever made me feel so powerful, so strong and so in touch with my body. I know that not everyone feels that way, and I know that a lot of women have complicated, traumatic births, but just keep an open mind when it comes to your own birth. There's no predicting how it will turn out, and you might be surprised how much you enjoy it.

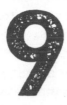

WELCOME TO BABYGEDDON

Having just read Chapter 7 about the physical aftermath of giving birth, you may be thinking, jeez Louise, that's a lot to deal with. And you're not wrong, it really is. However, the postpartum fun doesn't end with your ragged bits.

As if navigating cracked nipples, a swollen bumhole and a tsunami of uterine lining falling out of your vagina wasn't enough, there's also the small issue of your emotional and mental wellbeing to contend with. Becoming a mum for the first time is a MASSIVE life-changing experience, but it's easy to underestimate just how challenging the transition into parenthood can be. For a lot of new mums, myself included, the first few months can be – now, how do I put this delicately? – a bit of an emotional shitshow. It's a highly charged time with heightened emotions that are fuelled by a discombobulating concoction of hormonal changes, a huge lifestyle adjustment and extreme sleep deprivation. Frankly, it's a lot to process.

Over the next few pages, I will highlight just some of the emotions new mums may experience in the midst of the early postpartum haze, and explore some of the challenges that can arise out of the experience. From grappling with the absence of an immediate overwhelming rush of love for your baby, to feelings of entrapment and being overwhelmed due to the reality of being on call 24/7 to fulfil the needs of a tiny, milk-guzzling sleep thief. Not to mention the mind fuck of solving the basic practicalities of looking after a baby and then dealing with all the fears and worries that you're getting everything wrong because you have NO IDEA WHAT YOU'RE DOING!

Hopefully you will finish this chapter with an insight into what to expect emotionally during the first few months of new parenthood, alongside some helpful advice and suggestions for surviving it. Of course, some of you will sail seamlessly into your new role singing 'Kumbaya' and shooting rainbows out of your vagina. But for those of you who don't, if you do experience any of the following, just know that you aren't alone and that having a hard time and not relishing every second of the endless nappy changes, night feeds and general delirium induced by sleep deprivation does not make you a bad mum. It just makes you human.

Mama's got the blues

As we've previously explored, pregnancy and birth involve a dick load of hormones, with oestrogen and progesterone playing the most pivotal role of all. O&P, as I'm affectionately going to call them, are known as steroidal hormones and are key to creating dopamine and serotonin, two neurotransmitters in the brain that are integral to feeling calm and happy. Studies have shown that this dynamic duo also influence the areas of our brain that regulate mood, behaviour and cognitive abilities. Basically, they're pretty essential in making us feel emotionally and mentally balanced, and when they get out of whack you can end up feeling like utter shite.

While you are pregnant O&P will be at the highest levels your body will ever experience, but they take a rapid nose dive as soon as your placenta (the source of said elevated hormone levels) is delivered. This dramatic fall – a 1,000 per cent change in just a matter of days – allows your body to begin producing milk but it can also trigger the onset of extreme postpartum emotions.

Cue the baby blues! Now I'm sure a lot of you will have heard of this phenomenon, but guess what? Statistically speaking, the majority of you are going to experience it. It may not hit you straight away – in fact, the first 24 hours after labour can feel pretty damn euphoric for some women (thanks to all that oxytocin floating around from the birth), but it's estimated that 80 per cent of all mothers go through some form of postpartum emotional funk in the first few weeks after giving birth. And while baby blues may sound like a shade from the Farrow & Ball colour chart, it's far from being cutesy. Emotional Armageddon feels more appropriate, and it's all down to your hormones. This will look different for everybody, but expect to experience the following.

Your mood swings will take more twists and turns than the Big Dipper. Have you ever seen one of those massive fuck-off rollercoasters that makes your anus twitch with nervous anticipation just looking at it? You know the ones that dip and dive from the headiest heights to the lowest lows, and thrash the riders around like rag dolls, as they scream with sheer exhilaration combined with undertones of terror, through a series of unexpected twists and turns? You have? Good. Because riding the emotional waves of new parenthood is a bit like boarding the Big Dipper – it's fast, it's furious, it's full of extremes and it can hit you so hard that you come out the other end thinking 'what the fuck just happened?' It's helpful to remember that your emotions are magnified during this period, so try not to stress that you'll always feel this unstable, because you won't. Just take each day at a time and embrace whatever you're feeling in the moment, good or bad.

You'll feel like a big fat Debbie downer. Having a baby is supposed to be the most joyous event of your life, right? Then how come you feel so bloody sad? Again, this is down to the drop in progesterone messing with your pleasure receptors, but feeling this way can be disconcerting, especially if you've never suffered from depressive feelings before. And that bummed-out feeling may not be helped by the challenging realities of new motherhood. Breastfeeding might be a nightmare, you probably won't be getting any sleep and you still can't take a shit without feeling like your perineum is going to burst open. All of this can come as a bit of a shock and leave you feeling at a lower ebb than your postpartum titties will eventually hang, so it's no surprise that you're struggling to find the joy in parenthood right now.

You may find yourself crying A LOT during these spells of sadness, and sometimes over the tiniest, most seemingly insignificant events. Even something as basic as burning the toast can activate the waterworks and leave you in the crux of an existential crisis. And the strangest part is that once the tears start, you may find it impossible to switch them off! They flow and flow out of your face like hot salty streams of emotion until your tear reserves literally dry up and your eyes are left feeling like two shrunken raisins. So get the tissues ready, babe, you'll need them.

You'll be worried about EVERYTHING. You may never have experienced anxiety before, or on the opposite end of the scale, you'll be a seasoned stress head, but suddenly you're plagued by a sense of impending dread and feel restless, panicky and constantly worried. What if something happens to the baby? What if you aren't doing this right? What if your partner leaves you because all you do is cry? What if you aren't capable of being a mother? ARGHHHHH! The cycle of doubts and fears plays round your brain like a broken record and you find yourself fretting over every little thing.

This can be particularly challenging if you tend to err on the side of perfectionism, because, babes, if you think you're going to be able to micro-manage a newborn, you can't. Nothing goes to plan, there's very little schedule and you have to accept that your baby can't be pigeon-holed into your expectations. Just relinquish control.

You'll be consumed with burning rage. I'm not sure this emotion is talked about freely, maybe because most mums are afraid to admit it, but it's perfectly normal to be filled with the wrath of Satan in these early days after delivery. Whether it's being angry at yourself for not knowing how the fuck to mother this tiny human, being mad at the world because your baby won't stop crying or, most likely, feeling inexplicable animosity towards your partner for not being the one having to deal with all this mothering bullshit, stuff just pisses you off.

The highlight of my fury was sitting across the room feeding Oliver in the middle of the night and staring at my other half as he slept. The indignation and outrage I felt towards him not having to wake up every forty-five minutes and having his nipples ravaged by a newborn could well have led to violence. I was so jealous of his freedom and autonomy, and just sat there thinking what an absolute bastard he was for not having to endure the same shit as me. This was, in fact, a big motivator for choosing to combi-feed our second child, so we could share the nights and I wouldn't be wishing him dead every night. If we hadn't gone down that feeding route, I reckon I would be writing this book from prison.

You'll find it difficult to switch off. This one feels like a total kick to the tits when you're already exhausted, but lots of new mums will experience temporary insomnia postpartum and find falling asleep and staying asleep much more challenging. So if your baby waking 17,484,792 times a night doesn't succeed in keeping you awake, your hormones will. WHY, MOTHER NATURE? WHY?! Yet again this is down to the decrease in the production of progesterone (it has sleep-inducing properties), as well as changes in levels of melatonin, which the body produces in the evening to promote sleepiness and relaxation. These adjustments can affect your circadian rhythm, which regulates not only sleep but also mood, appetite and other bodily functions. Couple this with your new mate anxiety keeping your brain busy catastrophising shit, and it's a miracle new mums get any shut eye at all!

You'll feel incredibly vulnerable. It's no surprise that dealing with this onslaught of erratic emotions is going to leave you feeling vulnerable. Being a nutjob is exhausting. Especially when it's accompanied by feeling physically compromised on account of the forty-two stitches holding your vagina/stomach together. You're going to feel a teeny-weeny bit defenceless. What you really need now is someone to scoop you up, give you a big cuddle, let you sleep for 48 hours and reassure you that everything is going to be OK. So, babe, EVERYTHING IS GOING TO BE OK! And it might not just be you reeling from reality of looking after a newborn. Your partner might be struggling with the adjustments too (although you always win the 'who's more fucked up?' award, so don't worry). However bleak it feels in the pits of the postpartum funk, things will get better.

For most women, thankfully this emotional disruption is temporary and shouldn't last longer than approximately six weeks. By three months postpartum, oestrogen and progesterone levels should return to pre-baby levels, and by six months, your body should have come full circle and you'll be feeling (almost) completely back to normal. It's not a case of the baby blues passing within a couple of days or weeks; it's going to take you a good few months to feel back to your old emotionally well-balanced self, and that is perfectly OK.

If you experience any of these emotions for a prolonged period of time or they feel so overwhelming that they interfere with your day-to-day life, it could be an indicator of postpartum depression. One in five women will develop mental health problems during pregnancy and in the first year after childbirth, but many women don't seek help, believing these emotions are just part and parcel of having a baby. Obviously there is a difference between the baby blues and postpartum depression, so being aware of what is expected at this stage, versus what could be a sign of a bigger problem, is critical to seeking diagnosis and treatment as soon as possible. It's very helpful if you, your partner and your family read about the symptoms so that if you do become unwell, you realise what's happening and seek professional help. I've provided a list of symptoms to look out for below.

Postnatal depression and anxiety

I've talked at length about the kaleidoscope of emotions you can feel during the postpartum period, but for some women, feelings of depression, low mood and anxiety aren't simply down to the baby blues. Signs that you or someone you know might be suffering from postpartum depression (PND) include:

- A persistent feeling of sadness and low mood.
- Lack of enjoyment and loss of interest in the wider world.

- Lack of energy and feeling tired all the time.
- Trouble sleeping at night and feeling sleepy during the day.
- Difficulty bonding with your baby.
- Withdrawing from contact with other people.
- Problems concentrating and making decisions.
- Frightening thoughts – for example, about hurting your baby.

Like any other form of depression, PND can impact every aspect of your life, affecting your relationships, your self-esteem and confidence, your health and the bond you have with your baby. If you notice that you're feeling any of the above, contact your GP or healthcare provider and reach out for help.

Once diagnosed, postpartum depression can be treated with medication and talking therapy. You do not have to suffer alone.

No rest for the wicked ... or the new mum

Now we've covered how your hormones can dick about with your equilibrium, let's take a look at the mind-boggling effects of sleep deprivation. As soon as your baby arrives, the concept of time will no longer be applicable to your life. 'What do you mean?!' I hear you cry. 'Keeping time is the basis of my entire existence!' Yep. As it is for all of us ... except babies!

Newborns operate in their own unique time zone that bears absolutely no correlation to the time-keeping management systems that you and I are so accustomed to conforming to. They do not give a shit whether it's 10a.m. or 10p.m. and pretty much just sleep and feed whenever the fuck they want to.

We're going to delve much deeper into your baby's sleep needs in a couple of chapters, but to give you a rough idea of what to expect; for the first few weeks at least, most babies will operate on roughly a 2–3 hour feeding schedule AROUND THE CLOCK, and then take anywhere between 20–45 minutes to do the actual feeding. This feels manageable in the daytime but maybe not so groovy at night when you're woken up every couple of hours by a hungry baby needing a feed. Now if you're bottle or combi-feeding, you won't have to take this hit alone as you can share the load with your partner. But if you're exclusively breastfeeding, then, babes, you're going to be existing on very little sleep. I mean, who needs sleep anyway, right? It's not like you were in labour for sixteen hours and have used every ounce of your physical and mental energy to get a baby out of your womb. Or that doing so has left you feeling like you've run eight marathons and your pelvic floor is about to flop out. Oh, wait a minute …

It seems a very cruel blow that after the sheer exertion of birth, our selfish sleep-sabotaging babies don't even give us the opportunity to get one night of uninterrupted sleep to recover. And that's just the beginning! A couple of nights of broken sleep and your brain will be fried from exhaustion.

Now if you've never experienced extreme sleep deprivation and, like me, you have the sleep needs of a sloth, this interruption to your normal routine can really take its toll on the old noggin. Neuroimaging and neurochemistry studies suggest that a good night's sleep helps foster both mental and emotional resilience, while chronic sleep deprivation sets the stage for negative thinking and emotional vulnerability. Just what you need when your hormones are already running riot.

After a few weeks of surviving on broken snippets of sleep, you can feel that you're living in an alternate reality where time really has no meaning and the days just roll into one endless, surreal blur. You may find yourself experiencing low mood or feeling hyper-emotional, anxious and inexplicably pissed off – and that your cognitive functioning and performance are affected. Forgetfulness, making mistakes and slower thinking than normal are all common side-effects of extreme tiredness. I can only liken it to feeling that your brain has been replaced with a bowl of mashed potato. I would constantly forget what I was in the middle of, would struggle to form coherent sentences and would do curious things like put the oven gloves away in the freezer and my toothbrush in my knicker drawer. It felt like all the wires in my brain that enabled me to function had been yanked out and then clumsily shoved back in the wrong holes. Which only served to make me feel even more vulnerable and believe I was losing my mind.

At my most sleep-deprived, I was woken by my baby for a feed, pulled him to my chest to breastfeed, thought I'd latched him to my tit but then couldn't work out why I could still hear crying. It took me a good few confused minutes to realise that I had in fact picked up a pillow and was trying to tenderly breastfeed it, leaving my baby still lying there desperately searching for my nipple.

In a funny way, you do adjust to the broken sleep, and whereas once only getting four hours of consecutive shuteye a night would have felt like torture, with a newborn it feels as restorative as a weekend break at a spa. Ultimately you can't force your baby into a routine just yet, so you're going to have to ride out this sleep-deprived mayhem as best you can. My advice in these first few weeks is to rest at every goddamn given opportunity you get. Take naps, stay horizontal in bed with your baby, don't make grand plans, let go of how tidy your house is and keep visitors to an absolute minimum (see 'Self-care tips').

And just to give you hope, there is good news. Sleep should begin to naturally improve around the 2–3 month mark as your baby's circadian rhythm begins to regulate between day and night and they sleep for longer stretches. So although you feel like the sleepless nights and the eyes like piss holes in the snow will never end, have hope that at some point they will. And while you wait, follow my sleep-deprivation survival tips in Chapter 11 on page 227.

Just let me poo in peace

So we've discovered how integral sleep and hormonal balance are to feeling like a sane, functioning human, but what emotions can arise from the inevitable lifestyle changes your baby will bring? 'What do you mean lifestyle changes?' I hear you exclaim. 'Our baby won't have an impact on our lifestyle! We fully intend to do all the wonderful things we did BEFORE having kids!' HAHAHA! Good luck with that one, babes.

Now I'm not saying that it isn't possible to lead the lifestyle you did pre-kids (I am), I'm just warning you that kids make doing anything spontaneous, fun and carefree a lot more complicated. Impromptu brunches, weekends away with friends, lazy Sundays frolicking in bed, lie-ins … GONE. When there's a small human to cater for, the focus is well and truly off you, babes – from now on everything revolves around them. Even the mundane everyday tasks that you would never have consciously considered, now become a complex operation that requires thought and planning to ensure you can feed/comfort/attend to your baby at any given moment if you need to.

Doing a poo, for example. Before kids, you probably never gave it a thought, right? Just felt your sphincter twitch, dropped your keks and curled out a turd no problems. And I bet you got to read a book or scroll Instagram for 20 minutes while doing it. LUCKY BASTARD. Now let's fast-forward to the same scenario but with the responsibility of looking after a newborn baby. You feel a tremor in your bumhole, but the baby is screaming and you can't put them down, so you have to suck up your turtlehead and crack on. Twenty minutes later and the urge comes again but now you're in the middle of a feed with a baby attached to your tit so yet again, you clench your cheeks and crack on with your duties. Now two hours and three strong coffees later since initially needing this shit, your body can't take it any more – you're touching cloth and one way or another, this poo is coming out. But guess what, you're in the middle of another fucking feed. Rather than shit yourself, you decide to make a dash to the bog, bringing the nipple nibbler with you. And there you find yourself, sitting on the toilet with faeces flowing out of you while a baby suckles your areolas, wondering how on earth you're going to manage to wipe your bum one-handed without covering both of you in poo. Work out the logistics of that one!

This will all become second nature after a couple of weeks, and pretty soon shitting with a baby latched on your nork will be the norm. But initially, the starkness of how drastically different your life has become with a baby in tow can throw up all sorts of abstruse emotions. You may feel overwhelmed by your new responsibilities and having to keep a tiny baby's needs met around the clock 24/7. You may feel trapped and suffocated by the lack of autonomy over your body and your freedom. You may miss your old life and wish that you could just fuck everything off and have one blissful day all to yourself. And if you feel all that, then inevitably you'll feel immense guilt and failure for even entertaining these thoughts and emotions in the first place.

Confronting these feelings can be uncomfortable, especially when our preconception of motherhood is so idealised. Remember the influence that media, film and TV has on our understanding of birth? Well, motherhood is much the same. It's all picture-perfect scenes of rosy cheeked babies, who never cry, being cradled by impeccably turned out mothers with beaming smiles, and not a hint of rage or sadness or a single sick-stained shoulder in sight. So when the reality hits that your kid won't stop screaming, you haven't showered in two days, you can't stop crying and your thighs are chafed from the wings of your massive sanitary towel, it's not surprising that we feel we're the ones doing something wrong and failing. But the fact is, new parenthood is fucking brutal.

Your life will feel so drastically different from how it was pre-baby and it's OK to find that a challenge. Mothering is not instinctive for everyone, and even if it is, it takes time to nurture and some of us have to learn on the job and work really bloody hard to master it. That is absolutely OK and not a reflection of your ability to mother. And let's not forget that you're having to deal with all this on top of wildly fluctuating hormones, extreme sleep deprivation and still in physical recovery from birth. So yeah, let's scrap that fantasy of motherhood, give ourselves a bloody break! The transition to motherhood is a tough one.

A word from Rob

I was rather shocked the first time I read this chapter. Victoria and I have always had an open and honest relationship and have been able to talk about anything – or at least that's what I thought. I was aware it wasn't all sunshine and rainbows after Oliver arrived, due to Victoria crying as much as she did. Especially as I'm the one normally sobbing at a rom-com while she's sitting stony faced. However, she kept it from me that she was finding it hard to love our new arrival and just how much she was struggling mentally. I've since learned she felt like a failure, as if something was wrong with her and she was too ashamed to admit that to me. So you need to be prepared for your partner to possibly be feeling some of these emotions. Try to get her talking about how she is feeling – if you are like me, this can be a challenge, as usually after the fourth 'y'alright love?' in a row she looks ready to punch me in the face. My tactic when she was really low was to call someone that I knew she trusted and who she could open up to. Her mum. I would call Trish and tell her that I thought Victoria was struggling and ask her to give her a call, and this really worked.

I personally found the first month pretty crazy; everything is all so new and intense and you've likely not experienced sleep deprivation like this before – unless you've completed Royal Marine Commando hostage training. I was lucky in that I got two weeks' paternity leave and I added another two weeks' leave to that so I could be around. If you are privileged enough to be able do the same, I would definitely recommend it.

But what will I be doing, I hear you ask? You need to be there to provide emotional support to your partner, but also to give her a break from the baby whenever possible. This is also your time to bond with the baby, get in all those cuddles, skin-on-skin time, baby massages, looking into their eyes, listening to their funny baby noises. I enjoyed singing and reading to them as well. Then you need to get stuck in on that nappy changing (first-month poo is gross and incredibly varied), cooking, cleaning the house, bringing your partner regular food and drinks, attending breastfeeding support groups with her, and fending off well-wishers who want to descend on you straight away.

The last point is especially important ... First time round we welcomed guests almost immediately and we really weren't ready for it. We were both delirious from sleep exhaustion, and Victoria was physically and emotionally depleted, neither of which are ideal for entertaining, especially when some family members are challenging at the best of times. So really think about if you are up for it, and if not, feel no shame in telling your family to give you all some space until you're ready.

I managed to gather a small mountain of what I like to call 'negative Brownie points' during Victoria's pregnancy, and unfortunately if you are not able to share some of the burden of feeding the baby then you will be racking up even more of these bad boys post-birth. The eldest has just celebrated his fifth birthday in a sweaty, overcrowded soft play centre, and I am still up to my eyeballs in brownie-point debt. If your partner is breast-feeding, prepare for death stares from across the room every night – minus ten points each time. The fact that you will also be getting disturbed sleep and feeling horrendous apparently doesn't count for anything if it's not your nips being chewed on. This was the situation with our first child, despite my protests that we should get some formula so I could help out and she could take a much-needed break. Back then Victoria was convinced by the 'Breast is Best' admittedly alliterative and catchy sloganeering, despite it damaging her mental health, her relationship with the baby and her areolas. If the mum has decided not to exclusively breastfeed, volunteer for as many feeds as she will accept so she can get the sleep she desperately needs to recover from the birth. Combi-feeding our second child meant I was able to do this – clawing back a few points – and this came with the added benefit that I bonded with the baby much more in those first months than I had when I wasn't involved in feeding our first.

Also be prepared for your partner to hate you with every fibre of their being once you return to work. It doesn't matter that you were nose-deep in a stranger's armpit on the commute, your boss tore you a new one for not submitting the accounts on time and you got stuck being talked at by tedious Graham from HR about his golfing weekend, she could still be annoyed that you got a 'break' and curse you for it. So play down work chat when you get home, and don't be a prick and accept every (or any) post-work drinks invite that comes your way.

Partner pep talk

If ever there was a time that your partner needs you, it's now. Sure, she was vulnerable during pregnancy and labour, but this is the moment you need to step up and prop up that bitch like you've never propped her up before. Non-negotiable ways you can support her are:

- Reading this chapter to get an insight into everything she's going to be feeling.
- Taking over the domestic duties. I'm talking washing/ cleaning/cooking/changing the bed sheets/emptying the bins – and all without being prompted.
- Making sure she's hydrated – it's good for recovery and if she's breastfeeding she'll need the extra fluid.
- Checking she's comfortable – imagine pushing an orange out of your bellend. It's going to sting, right? Of course it is, so make sure you've got plenty of pain relief, ice packs and cushions on hand for whenever she needs them.
- Letting her express all her emotions with no fear of judgement.
- Looking out for the signs of postnatal depression.
- Supporting her feeding decisions – if it's not your tits involved, you really have no say.
- Giving her reassurance and encouragement when she feels like a pile of shit.
- Limiting guests.
- Taking the baby so she can rest/sleep/have some alone time.

- Never referring to looking after the baby as you 'babysitting'. It's your fucking baby too, mate.
- Not organising a night out with the lads four days after the baby is born (unless you want your balls cut off).

Light at the end of the tunnel of turmoil

Writing this chapter has brought back memories of my own intense emotional experience of becoming a mum for the first time, and reminded me just how much I struggled in those early days. I think there's often so much emphasis on pregnancy and giving birth when you're expecting a baby, that the small matter of what happens post-delivery is somewhat overlooked. This might go some way to explain why it can come as such a massive shock, and why a lot of new mums are left feeling like a rabbit in the headlights, totally over-whelmed by the reality of it all.

In all honesty, I wonder how the fuck I ever survived the brutality and rawness of those first few weeks. Alongside the physical fallout of birth, breastfeeding struggles and (barely) surviving on about twenty minutes of consecutive sleep a night, I was a bit of a wreck. I had no idea what I was doing, I felt completely exhausted, burnt out, alone and scared and like my body was failing me and there was absolutely nothing I could do about it. Not to mention the doubt, the guilt and the feelings of suffocation and entrapment that come with being solely responsible for the life of a tiny person. And on top of that, I felt no real connection to this snuffling creature who literally gnawed my areolas until they bled and just cried and cried and kept me awake all night. It was carnage. I'm pretty sure I Googled 'am I a shit mum?' and 'how do you love a baby?' about 18,548,320 times because, honestly, despite us being sold this idea that women are natural mothers, I felt so far from that I just wanted to up and run away. Of course that feeling faded with time, and after about six months I woke up one morning and it didn't feel like my mind was swimming through hot tar.

We underestimate the impact becoming a parent has on our mental health and I just wish I'd known that I wasn't the only one who felt completely fucked up on becoming a new mum. That is why I feel this chapter is so integral to this book. I hope that reading this leaves you feeling a little more prepared and a little less overwhelmed if you do indeed have a similar experience to me and the thousands of other new mums who have struggled to make sense of their new role.

The mental load of new parenthood may leave you questioning what has happened to your life, how you will cope and whether the mayhem will ever end. But you'll be pleased to hear that despite the carnage of the first few months, things do get easier and one day you'll look back at this time and commend yourself for getting out of it in one piece. It's fucking tough, but no matter how dark the days get, or how little you believe in your own capabilities to mother, there is help and support out there if you need it. Whether it's talking to your partner, calling your kids twats with your bestie or seeking professional help – whatever makes the mental load of motherhood lighter, do it. You are not a bad person for not relishing every second of parenthood but, most importantly, you are not alone.

Self-care

Looking after yourself and your baby while dealing with the absolute shitshow of new parenthood can feel impossible. Lots of new mums do not give themselves the time and space they deserve just to heal and adjust to their new life, but I'm here to tell you that you are allowed to give yourself a break. Self-care is probably further down your list of priorities than giving your partner a blowic right now, but make it one! I'm not talking spa days here, hun, I'm talking simple, achievable steps to staying sane and looking after yourself. Here are my top tips for preserving your emotional and mental wellbeing.

Guests

When your baby is born, your family and friends are going to want to visit immediately. This is lovely in theory, but in reality guests can actually be a bit of a pain when all you really need is rest. Personally, I would limit guests to an absolute minimum and be selective. Ask yourself, what will 'insert family member name here' bring to the table?

If Aunty Sandra wants to drop round a week's supply of lasagne and then insists on doing the washing up, she's welcome! But if Uncle Nigel is going to expect YOU to make HIM a brew despite the fact you have a gigantic grapefruit of a haemorrhoid hanging out of your arse, he can fuck right off. Might seem a bit harsh refusing people who want to come round, but honestly, babies are boring anyway so they won't be missing out. And if they do have to come round, put a time limit on their visit so it's short and sweet.

The domestic load

It's safe to say that your house is probably going to end up looking like a bit of a shit tip in these first few months of parenthood. Well, actually forever now that you have kids. As hard as it is to let go of the domestic chores like cleaning, shopping, washing, cooking, if you can let your standards slip during these first few months and lower your cleanliness expectations, you probably won't feel as frustrated about having a messier house than you usually like.

I also think this is the perfect opportunity for your partner to get stuck in and take total control of domesticity. Haha, I hear the seasoned mums cry, good luck with that one! But I'm serious. They can shop, cook and clean and you do as little as possible, love, and don't feel guilty about it. Pretty soon your baby slug will be wide awake demanding your attention, so take advantage of the fact that this little sproglet isn't going to be doing much for a while and CHILL your sewn-up flaps.

Keep plans to a minimum

In a lot of cultures, new mums are practically ordered to have bedrest for the first six weeks after birth. But here in the UK it seems that there's an expectation that life will go right back to normal as soon as your baby is born. We want to be out for lunch, doing baby classes, meeting friends, going to frigging exercise classes. All that stuff is great, but honestly, there's no rush to get back into the swing of things immediately if you don't want to.

Doing too much and making too many commitments too soon can actually lead to you feeling more burnt out and exhausted than you realise. I'm not saying be a fucking hermit, I'm just saying that all this lovely stuff can come later on, when your body and mind are a bit further into recovery. Don't do what I did and embark on a stupidly long walk two days after giving birth and end up by the side of the road hyperventilating with panic because I thought my uterus was going to fall out on to the pavement. Get back into bed!

However, the benefit of having a newborn is that they are relatively easy and portable and you're not yet a slave to their nap schedule, so if you want to get out there and be a part of the real world outside your newborn bubble, do it. Your bed will also be waiting for you when you get home.

Practise mindfulness

Remember how I banged on about the power of Barry the sex-pest breath earlier? Well, guess what, Barry and his sexual deviancy need resurrecting right now. Studies have shown that mindful meditation and associated breathing techniques can lower heart rate, reduce blood pressure and calm the sympathetic nervous system – making them excellent tools for nurturing your emotional and mental wellbeing. And you don't have to go all tantric spiritual guru to reap the benefits, just five minutes a day will do the job.

Taking care of your needs

We hear the terms 'self-care' and 'me time' bandied around loads these days but what does that really mean when you're a new mum? Taking a bubblebath and lighting a scented candle? Nah, mate, that's not what we're talking about here. You don't have to be getting an Indian head massage for it to qualify as self-care. It's about looking after the small things – like being able to take a shit by yourself, eat a proper meal, have a nap when you need it – that all adds up to making you feel less like a chaotic mentalist.

I know taking time for yourself may seem totally impossible with a newborn, especially if you're breastfeeding and need to be around to feed the baby. But you will start to see a pattern to your baby's sleep/feeding needs and can factor in some pockets of time for you while they're sleeping. On a very basic level, fulfilling your need to get washed, dressed and fed will keep you feeling connected to some semblance of normality. Some days it'll all go to shit and you'll still be sitting in your pjs at 4p.m., but when you can, give that minge a rinse and get a sandwich down your gob.

And carving out the space to be alone, no matter what you're doing, can do wonders for restoring your sense of self. Even a quick trip to Tesco to browse the clothes aisles by yourself can feel like the most exciting and liberating time of your life. But having that time away, albeit brief, is an opportunity to reset, gain some autonomy and remember what it feels like just to be you without a baby hanging off you.

And don't fall into the seductive lull of aimlessly scrolling social media when you find yourself alone. It'll eat up your time while offering very little reward, and nine times out of ten, it will also leave you feeling more shit than you did before. Save it for the 40-minute breastfeeds when there's literally dick all else to do.

Ask for help

This is probably the most essential piece of advice in this list. Do not, for one minute, think that you have to suffer anything alone in this crazy journey. Whether it's needing support from your partner, hiring a breastfeeding consultant, talking to your doctor about postnatal depression or simply offloading how you're feeling to a friend, don't be afraid to be open and honest about what you're feeling and asking for help if you need it. It doesn't make you a failure or a bad mum and it could make a huge difference to your wellbeing.

Whatever you need help with – the domestic chores, making nutritious meals that encourage your milk supply, wanting to know if it's normal to hate your partner, how to ease colic, how to combat sore nipples or any other number of random questions you have – talk about it all! If you made friends through your antenatal group, whack it on a WhatsApp group, go on parenting forums, discuss it with your partner, ask your mum/best friend/woman sitting next to you on the bus – someone, somewhere has been through it all before, but you'll never find out until you ask.

And if it's specialist help you need, there is a whole host of postpartum experts out there ready to help. From lactation consultants to cranial osteopaths, to postpartum nutritionists – if you need help for a specific problem, get on Google and find someone who can help you. You never, ever have to suffer alone.

The silver lining in the bag of dicks that motherhood has handed you

Now I couldn't write this chapter without including a sliver of hope amongst all this emotional turmoil. Thankfully, new parenthood does have wonderful moments of unadulterated bliss and happiness – and thank god! If it didn't, I don't think anyone would ever procreate again.

A big part of the reason you probably wanted to have kids in the first place was knowing they'd bring joy into your life, right? What you can't quite comprehend, perhaps, is just how fiercely that joy may manifest when your baby arrives. Things are about to get soppy, bitches, and I'm not talking about your leaky tits (although those too will be drenched from all the additional oxytocin jizzing round your body).

Despite newborns looking like miniature aliens and possessing the charisma of a slug – when you've spawned your own otherworldly mollusc, those minor details fade into insignificance. They can be boring as shit, look like Benjamin Button and literally have zero bants and you're still going to think the sun shines out of their tiny arse. Even your baby performing basic bodily functions like yawning, sneezing or dropping a ridiculously cute fart, can initiate a bout of insane jubilation and leave you either crying with happiness or in fits of euphoric giggles. Postpartum emotions are intensified by at least 100 per cent, so expect to get giddy. Just remember, though, Junior curling out his first turd might be the most beautiful and magical thing you've ever seen, but no one else gives a shit, love, so don't post it on Facebook.

When you're in the loved-up joyous zone, don't be surprised if you find yourself staring adoringly at your newborn for hours on end, taking in every detail of their little face and sniffing their head like a Labrador snuffling a bitch on heat. Inhaling a nostril full of your baby's scent actually initiates a neurochemical reaction in your brain and lights up your pleasure centres, much like getting a whiff of your favourite food or indulging in mind-altering drugs. So next time you fancy a bender, ditch the mushrooms and get a whiff of a baby instead.

Seeing as this is one of the few positive emotions I'm sharing in this chapter, I'm going to suggest that when you hit the joy zone, make the fucking most of it. Sniff that baby hard and soak up every inch of serotonin loveliness you can get, sister, and hopefully these moments of joy and happiness will be enough to carry you through all the other shit bits.

And if you find yourself completely devoid of joy, see 'Love at first sight' below and 'Postnatal depression' on page 190 for more help.

Love at first sight

From the moment I found out I was pregnant with my son, all I could think about was getting to meet my baby boy. Like many expectant mothers, I fantasised about our first precious moments together a million times over, and it always looked the same. I'd be shrouded in soft light, looking ethereal and majestic, the midwife would rise evangelically from between my legs, holding up my newborn baby like a prized gift from the gods, and then hand me his hot little vernix-coated body for our first embrace. I'd hold him in my arms, gaze down lovingly, our eyes would lock for the very first time and then – BANG! My heart would explode into a million pieces and every inch of my body would be flooded with a love so powerful, so intoxicating and so all-consuming that it would take my breath away. At long last, I'd be complete. Or so I thought.

The anticipation and excitement of finally meeting him in the flesh and getting to live out this fantasy kept me going through the shittiest bits of my pregnancy. The mental mood swings, the areolas like dinner plates, the grapefruit haemorrhoids – I knew it would all be worth it for the love I'd feel for him the second he was placed in my arms. Sound familiar? Because that's what we're told to expect, right? That every woman will fall unquestionably and resolutely head over heels in love with their baby the second it exits their vagina. It's a mandatory part of becoming a mother.

So imagine my surprise and my disappointment when the fireworks weren't there straight away. No instant bond, no overwhelming rush of love, just downright relief that there was no longer a gigantic head splitting my vagina in half. No one talks about the possibility that that connection may not be there immediately; there's an assumption that it just happens. But it's important to recognise that for some women those feelings of deep emotional attachment take time to nurture and won't surface until later on. And it's more important still to acknowledge that it's OK if that's the case for you. It doesn't make you a cold-hearted bitch, or a bad mum.

All sorts of shit can interfere with your emotions post-labour and impact your connection to your baby.

Maybe you had a difficult or challenging birth that left you feeling traumatised, maybe you were too off your tits on pain relief to know what was going on, maybe your baby needed intervention and was whisked away from you before you had the chance to embrace them, maybe breastfeeding was a disaster from the outset, or maybe they looked so different from the way you had imagined them, you just find it hard to connect. Or maybe there's no obvious explanation for feeling a disconnect but the whole experience of becoming a mother just feels like a surreal blur devoid of any identifiable feelings.

We are complex beings, with nuanced emotions, and it's not as simple as just automatically falling in love at first sight with your baby. This was certainly the case for me. I had a straightforward, unmedicated birth, everything was pretty textbook in terms of delivery and despite feeling overjoyed that my baby had arrived, I didn't get the rush of love I was expecting with either of my children straight away. It came much later, especially with my son. As I will explain in detail in the next chapter, breastfeeding him was a veritable shitshow fraught with complications and difficulties, and the torment of the experience most definitely impacted our relationship. But there was no real reason with my daughter.

First time round, not experiencing that initial outpouring of love left me bereft, feeling guilt and shame. I was too afraid to share my thoughts with anyone, even my husband, for fear that I'd be outed for being an absolute cunt who couldn't love their baby. I kept it a secret, wracked with feelings of inadequacy, failure and grief for not being the mother I thought I would be. None of this was helped by the fact that feeding him was sheer torture and with each painful feed I felt myself emotionally drifting further and further away from my baby. When we made the decision to stop breastfeeding at about three months in, the fog finally lifted. Slowly but surely our bond grew and I found it hard to believe that I'd ever struggled to love him. Pretty soon I was smitten, hook, line and sinker. Just as I described earlier in this chapter, I felt overwhelming joy to have this beautiful baby in my life.

When the same feelings of disconnect arose with my daughter, I wasn't worried. I knew that for me it would take a little longer to get there and I didn't beat myself up about it. Everyone's brain is wired differently and the way we foster emotional connection is completely unique, not to mention the impact that mental health can have on making those connections. Just rest assured that at some point, the floodgates will open and you will love your baby with such ferocity that you would literally kill for them if you had to.

10

BREASTFEEDING

Attack of the nipple-nibbling piranha

Of all the surprises that motherhood bestows upon you, the areola-busting reality of breastfeeding may be the most challenging. But breastfeeding is the most natural thing in the world, right? It's as simple as whacking out a tit, shoving a mouthful of areola into baby's mouth and, hey presto, your baby is feeding! Well, the truth is, while breastfeeding is a natural process, it doesn't necessarily come naturally for all of us. So although you may expect to breastfeed your newborn like a pre-Raphaelite goddess shrouded in sunlight and jizzing oxytocin out of your baps, you may discover that the reality is quite the opposite. Instead, breastfeeding may be more akin to Hieronymus Bosch's depiction of hell, where the endless nipple torture leaves you bedraggled and bereft, wailing like a banshee with a pair of red-raw, ravaged udders laid out like two undercooked ham hocks at an all-you-can-eat buffet. It can be carnage.

Of course, some women's areolas will take to breast-feeding like a pair of milky eager beavers. But for others, those first few days, weeks and even months of breast-feeding can be fraught with unexpected physical and mental challenges that feel incredibly overwhelming. Whether it's the literal pain of harbouring broken, bleeding nips, blocked ducts, mastitis or nipple thrush, or the existential struggle of having a tit limpet perma-nently attached to your chest, breastfeeding isn't necessarily a straightforward journey for everyone. And if it does end before you're ready, there's also the small matter of navigating the all-consuming shame and guilt that ensues from feeling your journey is ending prematurely.

But that's where this chapter should come in handy. Just think of me as your flappy fun-bagged fairy! Between my two sprogs, I've exclusively breastfed, exclusively pumped, combi-fed and exclusively formula-fed, so you could say I'm a bit of a feeding slag. I'm here to share my experiences of some of the complications and difficulties my titties faced, along with some practical advice of how to cope when your hooters end up looking like chewed-up luncheon meat. Plus I'll be sharing how you can keep your mental health in check, along with your bazookas, when both are left in tatters from the onslaught of breastfeeding. Some of the breastfeeding terminology I mention may already be familiar to you, but I hope you'll finish this chapter feeling prepared and equipped to take on any breastfeeding challenge, however it manifests. There's no doubt that breastfeeding is a beautiful experience, but the reality is, it can also be fucking brutal.

My milkshake brings all the babies to the yard

So first off, let's get to grips with the mechanics of breastfeeding. This is a very simple breakdown but it should give you a better understanding of how your milky norks function in the first few days and weeks after giving birth.

Much like labour, breastfeeding is a physiological process that relies on a combination of hormones being released in our brains to work. There are two hormones that directly affect breastfeeding: prolactin and our trusty old friend oxytocin. Put simply, prolactin helps your breasts to make the milk and oxytocin helps to get it out of you. Both are activated by the action of your baby suckling at your boobies, and the more you feed, the more milk you will produce.

Once your baby has exited your womb, you'll probably start worrying about when and how often you need to feed them. For the first feed, if you've had a straightforward, uncomplicated birth, your baby may feed either immediately or within a few hours of labour. Equally, they may be so knackered from having their head squashed through your vice-like vaginal canal that they need a big rest before contemplating taking a mouthful of areola. Either is fine, unless directed otherwise by the midwives. Babies need to feed little and often at the newborn stage, so from day one you'll probably be spending 80 per cent of your time with your tits out feeding your baby.

Generally, they will feed approximately every two to three hours, with each feed lasting anywhere from approximately 10 to 45 minutes on one or both tits. But just take that as a rough guide because every baby is different. General rule of thumb – or rather, tit – is that during this early phase you feed on demand whenever and wherever baby wants it. So it's up to you to learn their hunger cues and deliver their meals when they need them. Some hunger cues your baby may give to indicate it's dinner time include:

- Head turning or 'rooting' while eyeballing the room for titties.
- Fists moving to mouth and sucking on hands or lip-smacking.
- Trying to latch on to anything remotely nipple-shaped.
- Opening and closing mouth like a gormless goldfish.

As soon as they start showing signs that they're hungry, fill their gob. If your baby begins crying from hunger then it's likely you've missed these hunger cues. Crying is a late hunger signal and, if possible, we want to avoid it. However, it's easy to miss the early hunger cues in the brain fog of the early days of postpartum, so don't beat yourself up if it happens. You're new to this and it may take a little practice to hone your titty-feeding instincts.

In terms of what your hooters are up to once breast-feeding begins, your milk will be busy developing and adapting to the needs of your baby. The first stage of breast milk production consists of a thick, yellow, almost goo-like liquid, called colostrum, which is packed full of immune-boosting, growth-boosting and tissue-repair boosting goodness to help protect your baby. This then develops into a more mature, milk-like consistency around 3–4 days post birth. When this change occurs, production is well and truly established and it's like your boobs are suddenly flooded with liquid and the titty milk fountain is well and truly open. This process can be quite uncomfortable as your udders swell up like two overfilled water balloons fit to burst, but never fear, they will settle back down to less-gigantic proportions.

Most women find the first two weeks of breastfeeding particularly challenging as they get to grips with the logistics of breastfeeding, engorgement from the milk coming in and sore, cracked nips, plus all the other emotional bullshit that is going on with your postpartum mind and body. It's a bit rough, in all fairness. In theory, by approximately two weeks, your supply should start to settle down and feeding will become more comfortable. IN THEORY! By this point you might have had such a shit experience breastfeeding that you're ready to lob your tits off and put your baby on eBay. But we'll come to that!

OK, so let's talk about the physical act of breastfeeding. How the f do you achieve that? It's all well and good having this knowledge, but how do you actually get the little prick to feed from your ta-tas? Let's see if I can be of assistance.

Mastering the perfect positioning and attachment

In simple terms, positioning and attachment is how your baby connects to your breast. It's sometimes also referred to as 'the latch'. Master this and your baby will be awarded a golden ticket for permanent entry into the magical world of Titty Tonker's milk factory. Sign me up Tonker; sounds fantastic! In reality, this seemingly simple manoeuvre can sometimes feel as complex as having to solve a Rubik's Cube while blindfolded. Oh, and the Rubik's Cube is shaped like a nipple. It's easy to forget that although the physiological instinct for a baby to suckle is evolutionary, it doesn't necessarily mean they'll automatically attach to your breast effectively.

The biggest problem with trying to acquire this skill is the fact that we can't see what's happening in the baby's mouth when they're attached. Unable to methodically monitor our baby's milk intake, we instead have to rely on some form of mystical mother's intuition to determine what the fuck is actually going on. Which, funnily enough, is pretty difficult to muster when your body is still reeling from the very immediate trauma of having just extracted a human bowling ball from your uterus. Babies couldn't care less that you've been in labour for fourteen hours and need a week to recover, or that your insides are still slopping out of your minge like minced offal into your undercrackers – when they get hungry, you have to feed them. They're selfish bastards like that.

So how do you even start to master the perfect positioning and attachment? Those first couple of feeds will inevitably feel like a daunting task. You'll probably feel awkward, and clumsy and maybe even incapable – no thanks to the alarmingly flaccid nature of your baby's head flopping about at your tit like a strand of wet spaghetti. But it's OK – neither of you have done this before and it's going to be a learning curve for both of you. The basic aim here is getting enough areola into your baby's mouth to promote high milk flow and minimise nipple discomfort. Good positioning and attachment will ensure that both your nipple and a large portion of the areola are in the baby's mouth and it shouldn't hurt. I like to think of it as taking a bite out of a big juicy tit sandwich – you wouldn't lick the edges or suck the crusts, would you? No, you want to give your baby a big chunky mouthful of that delicious mammary panini.

Remember, achieving the optimum positioning and attachment is an acquired skill that takes time and practice to master, both for you and your baby, so it may take a while to get right. You'll know you're there when breastfeeding stops feeling uncomfortable or painful. This may happen within a few days or weeks, but for some women, it never feels quite right. So how do you know if your latch is lacking? Well, there are certain signs to look out for both for you and your baby. These include:

Baby

- Does not wake without being woken for feeds eight or more times in 24 hours.
- Latches on and off your breast frequently during feeding.
- Falls asleep within five minutes of latch-on.
- Does not suck regularly for the first seven to 10 minutes of a feed.
- Feeds for more than 30 minutes and is still hungry.
- Produces less than two poos in 24 hours by the end of the first week (for the first four to eight weeks).
- Produces fewer than six wet nappies in 24 hours by the end of the first week.

Signs of poor positioning and attachment for mum:
- Persistent sore or bruised nipples or areolas.
- Red, raw or cracked nipples.
- Creased or flattened nipples after feeds that look like they've been chewed.
- More than one episode of blocked ducts or mastitis.

If you or baby show any of these signs, get support from your midwife, GP or a breastfeeding consultant.

Fact is, some babies can't latch on as easily as others, some have problems staying awake to feed effectively, others have problems coordinating their suck, swallow and breathing patterns, and a few have conditions that affect the structure of the mouth that makes feeding difficult. Poor latch can occur for many reasons, but some of the most common are:

Being born prematurely. Babies do not normally learn to coordinate the sucking, swallowing and breathing needed for feeding until about thirty-four to thirty-six weeks of pregnancy. Put it this way, the smaller the gob, the more challenging it is to latch on. If they're born before this time, breastfeeding directly from the breast is not generally possible, but once they reach full term they should be able to master it.

How baby was delivered. During labour, baby's cranial bones move and overlap to pass through your vaginal canal – which explains why your newborn pops out with a cone head! This is normal and the bones usually return to their correct position over a few days after the birth, mostly via the process of the baby sucking. However, sometimes things don't return to normal and abnormal skull compression can affect your baby's feeding habits, including their ability to latch on. This is more likely to happen if you had a prolonged labour, your baby was born via emergency C-section, or forceps or ventouse were used during delivery. But luckily it can be corrected. I thoroughly recommend seeing a good chiropractor or cranial osteopath with expertise in treating newborn babies if this is your experience during birth. A couple of treatments can make a profound difference.

Tongue tie. When the *lingual frenulum* (the weird flappy bit of skin under your tongue that anchors your tongue to your mouth) is tight or short, it can impact how deeply your baby can latch on. Basically, the more your baby can extend their tongue and move it freely with a wide-open mouth, the more nipple they can guzzle into their gobs to feed. Some babies with a tongue tie breast-feed well from the start; others do so when positioning and attachment are improved. But any tongue tie that restricts normal tongue movement can lead to breast-feeding difficulties. Treatment is available in the form of a frenotomy – a simple procedure that divides the frenulum. You will need a referral from your GP or midwife, or you can seek private treatment for this.

Inverted or flat nipples. If your nips lack the girth for your baby to latch on to, it may be difficult for them to feed effectively. But it's not impossible! You can encourage your areolas to protrude by giving them a quick twiddle before feeding, gently pinching them to draw them out, and by wearing nipple formers – these are silicone discs that put gentle pressure on your nipples to draw them out in between feeds ready for dinner time.

Poor positioning. Finding the right feeding position where you feel comfortable and confident can really help to give baby the maximum areola-guzzling opportunity. There is a veritable Booby Sutra of nursing options out there; it's a case of trialling them and finding what works for you and your baby. And like any new skill, it takes practice, practice, practice! Some of the positions I favoured were cross-cradle, rugby ball, koala, side lying and upright, to name a few – in fact, I reckon I could have won the World Champion breastfeeding gymnastics with the positions I attempted. Much like my sex life, I personally favoured the laidback or nurturing position where you do just that, lie right back and let the other person do all the work. In the case of breastfeeding, you place baby tummy down on your chest and they wriggle their way to your nip and sort of bop on your tit like an inebriated woodpecker. It's minimum effort with maximum results and works really well with a newborn as it encourages a wide-open mouth, making that latch just a little bit easier. The only drawback is the practicality of finding a suitable place to lie down when you're out and about and the baby needs a feed – it's certainly not ideal down the frozen vegetable aisle in your local Tesco. That makes for a very awkward conversation with the security guard.

As mentioned previously, sometimes positioning and attachment just organically improve with time and practice, but sometimes it is also an indication that something else is going on that will require intervention.

BREASTFEEDING
203

Getting help

Breastfeeding support comes in lots of forms, but access-
ing it in the pits of breastfeeding hell may prove
challenging. Before baby arrives, do a bit of research and
have a list of breastfeeding contacts should you need to
seek help. If you attend an antenatal class, this is a good
place to start as they should be able to advise where you
can get support locally or even potentially offer it themselves. It's also worth investigating whether there's a
breastfeeding counsellor or lactation consultant attached
to your hospital before your baby arrives.

Generally, most areas have weekly local community
breastfeeding drop-ins, too, so while you still have half a
brain and you're getting longer than 45 minutes sleep a
night, write it down, stick it on the fridge and it'll be there
ready if things do go tits up. Of course, your midwife
should be able to support you in the first few days and
weeks after birth, as well as your health visitor. But in all
honesty, it's hit and miss as to their level of breastfeeding
expertise and helpfulness. Here are some of the other
breastfeeding professionals you may encounter:

Lactation consultant

The bee's knees of breastfeeding support, these tit wizards
are the Gandalfs of the boobing world. Generally, you have
to go private for the privilege of having one work their
milky magic on you, but their areola knowledge is infinite
and they will be able to assess even the most complex of
feeding issues. Assessments take place in person.

Breastfeeding counsellor

Next in the mammary ring are breastfeeding counsellors, aka the Aragorns of milk-making. These passionate pillow-pushers generally operate through breastfeeding charities and local breastfeeding groups but some hospitals also employ these lactating lushes. Most breastfeeding helplines are manned by breastfeeding counsellors, but it is also possible to book private consultations with them.

Mother-to-mother peer supporters

I coincidentally am one of these and you can think of us as the humble hooter hobbits. We've completed some basic breastfeeding training, we can offer emotional support but we can't make formal assessments and will signpost you to the appropriate channels when needed.

My only advice in engaging with any breastfeeding professional is to be aware that their views around breastfeeding may be quite rigid, with the mantra that breast is always best. That is what the training teaches you, but, as you have seen from my experience, it doesn't always work out that way. It's always worth doing your own research about breastfeeding as well as taking advice from professionals, but know that the important part of this journey is finding what works for you and your baby.

It has all gone tits up

For some of you lucky cows out there, by day four or five your milk will be flowing, you'll have found your preferred feeding position, baby will be nursing comfortably and you'll probably generally be feeling much more confident, albeit utterly exhausted. But for the unlucky cows out there, like me, at this point latching on may still be feeling about as comfortable as attaching a hungry piranha to your nips, and as appealing. If this is the case, something's probably not quite right. There are a whole host of issues that can arise from poor positioning and attachment; low weight gain, pain for longer than the first twenty seconds of a feed, damaged bleeding nipples, blocked ducts, a restless baby, baby coming off the breast repeatedly during feeds. The bottom line is, if baby doesn't get the milk it needs effectively during a feed, you're both going to end up royally pissed off, your nipples will feel savage and help will need to be sought. I wholeheartedly recom mend seeking additional support at this stage and have provided a handy guide in the Getting help information on the previous pages. There's no guarantee that they'll wave a magic booby wand and make everything better, but statistically speaking, the sooner you seek intervention, the greater your chance of maintaining breastfeeding.

When I hit difficulties feeding my son and was faced with the prospect of another harrowing feed, I took to the internet in a quest for the ultimate titting knowledge. I read every possible article going about how to position and attach your baby, watched countless videos of women dicking about with knitted tits and baby dolls on YouTube, Googled 'should my nipples be hanging off', and in my desperation, may have even asked my partner to 'just have a little go on them' to make sure my boobs were actually working. Our relationship has never been the same since.

My poor areolas had been shredded, they continuously bled and there was a friction blister the size of a testicle angrily pulsating on the tip of my right nipple. I became obsessed with watching Oliver feed, eyeballing each and every suckle and gulp with the fervour of a woman possessed and spunked money left, right and centre on creams, ointments, herbal aids, nursing teas, heat pads, cranial osteopathy – anything that could potentially ease the agonising ordeal of feeding him. I lost count of the number of strangers who ended up manhandling my malfunctioning norks. From the midwife, the GP, the health visitor to the lactation consultant, I had my puppies out more frequently than Jordan in her heyday.

Oliver was eventually diagnosed with a tongue tie (see above) and had it snipped, but by that point, the damage was done. Nothing helped. I felt hopeless, degraded, broken and most overwhelmingly that I had failed my baby. Looking back, I can see the impact that this experience had on my mental health but at the time I was so determined to stick to breastfeeding that it ended up being detrimental to my wellbeing. Not to mention the enormous impact it had on my bond with my baby. To be quite frank, I resented him. Being solely responsible for keeping him alive was suffocating and every time he started to cry I just wanted to run away with my broken tits forever.

Eventually, the combination of extreme sleep deprivation (at the worst point, I was surviving on stretches of only 45 minutes a night), the physical turmoil of having my norks ravaged continuously, day and night, and the crippling shame of inadequacy that I couldn't feed my baby, came to a head.

Dr Bumfluff saves the day

By week six, I was a total wreck. One night, after a feed that had lasted two long, arduous hours, I was sobbing on the bed, unable to put my pyjama top back on due to the unbearable pain of having anything against my flesh. My husband turned to me and gently whispered, 'Let's just give him a bottle.' I was enraged. A bottle? Of formula? How dare you! He may as well have said, 'Let's just give him some fucking anthrax'. I couldn't possibly give my baby that evil poison! The mere suggestion was an insult to my capability as a mother. Of course, I don't think that now; he just wanted to help me. He had witnessed my suffering daily and was genuinely worried about my wellbeing. But that didn't stop me from wanting to kick him in the balls. I fervently and foolishly resisted.

A few days later, I was back in A&E for the third time in so many weeks presenting with what looked like mastitis. The doctor on duty looked fresh out of puberty, never mind medical school. He had a patchy bumfluff beard, pimples and smelled distinctly of Lynx Africa. I went into the consultation room, unzipped my hoody and revealed one bright-red, gigantic, rock-hard nork. He went through the standard postpartum spiel you get in a medical setting; how many weeks is baby, how was delivery, how's feeding going, blah blah blah, but then looked up from his computer, stared directly into my eyes (which must have been difficult given the distraction of my massive tit) and tenderly asked, 'And how are you? Are you OK?'

Well, that was it. Through this whole process, having seen countless breastfeeding professionals, he was the first person to ask me how I was. The floodgates opened along with my infected udder. Tears started streaming down my face as I sobbed inconsolably and my hooter dripped warm milk into my lap like a leaky faucet. 'You can put your breast away now, Mrs Emes,' he pleaded. I wasn't doing very well, as a matter of fact I was doing fucking terribly. The weeks of pent-up frustration, sadness, disappointment, the dejection – it flowed out of me audibly like hot diarrhoea into a toilet pan. He leant over, placed his child-like hand on my arm and said, 'You're doing a brilliant job, but you know, you are allowed to stop. It's OK to just stop.' Whether it was his impeccable bedside manner or the intoxicating effect of his Lynx Africa, for the first time since starting breastfeeding, I felt seen. Of all people, this man-child understood my pain and I left that cubicle armed with a renewed faith in myself, determined to feed my baby, however that might manifest, free from my own unachievable expectations.

Tit troubles

Breastfeeding can throw up all sorts of issues, ranging from minor mammary niggles right through to serious complications that require medical treatment. Listed below are some of the more common tit troubles experienced by nursing mums and a few suggestions as to how to alleviate them.

Sore or cracked nipples

Now I don't think any breastfeeding mum is going to get away with never once having sore, cracked nipples. How could you?! Suddenly having a hot, wet, gummy mouth permanently encasing your areolas is going to take some getting used to. You may find the first few weeks particularly ravaging, with your areolas left feeling like they've had a cheese grater taken to them as opposed to a baby. The skin can become very sore and cracked, bleed and even form scabs. Delightful!

Back in the olden days, the general advice given to expectant mothers was to 'toughen' up their nipples prior to beginning breastfeeding. A number of methods were employed, from frequent rough nipple pinching and tweaking to administering vigorous areola rub-downs with abrasive materials. Women even suckled baby animals at their teats in a bid to harden their nipples. Don't worry, I'm not going to suggest whacking a kitten on your baps – these days we just treat sore nipples when they happen. THANK GOD.

Addressing the cause of the nipple soreness is the most effective way of solving it! Correcting positioning and attachment is paramount in allowing a damaged nipple to heal and enable pain-free, effective breastfeeding so should always be investigated. In the meantime, moist wound healing has been found to be the most effective way to heal a ravaged nip. Basically, this means keeping the area moist, either with a bit of expressed breastmilk or using lanolin creams and balms.

In my experience the only topical remedy that really helped were silver nipple shields. EXCUSE ME? These Madonna-esqe areola caps sit like little nipple hats in your bra and can be used in between feeds. They're the perfect tool for enabling moist wound-healing combined with a bit of expressed breast milk. Silver has healing, antibacterial and disinfectant properties, so it will give you immediate pain relief and help your skin to heal faster by protecting your nipples from contact with external bacteria.

For those in the trenches of sore nipples, a temporary solution may be nipple shields. Nipple shields are thin, nipple-shaped pieces of silicone that sit over your nipples as you feed. Using them is the equivalent of armouring up before entering battle – booby battle. They can help baby to get a deep latch, plus they provide a physical barrier between your breasts and their mouth, so they take some of the pressure off your battered nipples while nursing. Once baby has mastered the art of latching on and can easily deep-throat your nipples, you should be able to nurse without the shields. They're also helpful if you have a flat or inverted nipples as they tease your nipples out into two tiny erections.

Nipple shields are generally seen as a temporary solution, but some women rely on them for the duration of their breastfeeding journey. It's worth noting that there are downsides to using nipple shields as well as positives.

As it's harder for baby to get as much milk using nipple shields (20–25 per cent less milk than without), feeds can take much longer and baby may need topping up with expressed breast milk or formula after a feed. This may not be the case if your supply is bountiful, but for the majority of women, long-term use can impact their supply. This can be counteracted by doing more skin on skin with your baby. However, if it's the difference between trying them and it working for you or not trying them and your breastfeeding journey ending before you're ready, I'd say try them. But it may be worth seeking advice from a breastfeeding specialist or your midwife first.

If your nipples are so painful that you can't bear to feed, you can express instead. This gives your nips a break without disrupting your milk supply. Just express as frequently as you need to in order to mimic your baby's feeding pattern – so roughly every 2–3 hours until you feel ready to face the piranha again. If you do express, it's worth noting that your body may not respond in the same way it does to feeding your baby. Remember, breastfeeding is a physiological process and some women won't produce as much milk via a pump as they would via their baby. Just don't be disheartened if you pump and you get very little milk – it isn't necessarily a reflection of your supply. Expressing frequently is better than expressing for long periods of time. Generally, 20 minutes on both breasts should be long enough. If you struggle to express you can try doing your Barry sex-pest breath to relax (remember you need oxytocin to squirt), and covering your breasts so you can't see the milk coming out can also be helpful.

You can manage the pain of breastfeeding with paracetamol, ibuprofen and hot and cold compresses. Just remember that you shouldn't take painkillers continuously for longer than three days without consulting your GP. Painkillers can used to manage the pain temporarily, but if you're persistently in agony, seek intervention from a breastfeeding specialist.

Engorgement

Most mothers experience some engorgement in the first weeks after birth, especially when their milk comes in. Engorged breasts feel heavy, hard, warm and sensitive – like two giant testicles stuck on your chest desperate to deposit their load. When milk is removed, blood circulation improves and swelling reduces, so it's important you keep feeding or expressing.

You can reduce engorgement and swelling by using a combination of hot and cold compresses. Cold between feeds (frozen peas will do – and yes, you can refreeze them or, better yet, eat them) and warm compresses before feeding. Just apply moist warmth to your breasts for up to two minutes to help milk flow. Plus you can give your norks a good old rub-down and use gentle massage from the top of your tit down towards the nipple area in a circular motion.

Engorgement can lead to other breastfeeding problems, such as blocked ducts and mastitis, so get massaging as soon as you feel uncomfortable.

Blocked milk ducts

One of the side-effects of a poor latch is the breast not being drained properly, which can lead to complications such as blocked milk ducts and mastitis. Skipping feeds, a tight bra or awkward sleeping positions are also culprits. You'll know you've got a blocked duct when your breast resembles a rock in your nursing bra, feeling hard and painful. It might also be red, warm to the touch and slightly tender. Normally you can feel a localised lump in your breast where the blockage has occurred.

As soon as you realise you're harbouring a nobbily concrete nork, you will need to work on unblocking it. You can take ibuprofen for the inflammation, alternate hot and cold compresses on the affected area, place fridge-chilled Savoy cabbage leaves in your bra, express, try to feed through the agony and lube that bowling-ball titty up for the longest, firmest, stroke-heavy massage of its life – it brings a whole new meaning to the term tit wank. The vibration from an electric toothbrush applied to the area is also thought to help.

If the lump has not cleared after a day or two, or symptoms worsen (you develop a fever and flu-like symptoms), see your GP, as it may have progressed to mastitis.

Mastitis

Mastitis is a brutal step up from a blocked duct. It normally occurs in one breast, which becomes red, hot and painful, and it normally requires antibiotic treatment. It's also accompanied by flu-like feelings and often a temperature.

Alongside a swollen tit, you may notice that your baby is reluctant to feed from the breast affected. This is due to the sodium content in your milk rising and some babies don't like the taste of a salty nork. If you've never experienced the joy of housing a blocked duct the size of a golf ball, just imagine that your tit is taking a monumental beating with a rusty nail-adorned baseball bat while getting set alight with a flamethrower. Then throw in feeling that your blood is moving through your veins like tar, your entire body aches and your brain is being squeezed in a vice ... that should hopefully give you an inkling of just how FUCKING painful this bullshit is.

My advice for coping with this fiery fun-bag-busting beast? Employ all the pain-relieving techniques as described above, try to keep feeding or expressing to keep the milk flowing, but also call your doctor immediately. Mastitis can worsen rapidly if left untreated, resulting in an abscess, and in the worst-case scenario, develop into sepsis. If it gets to this point you would need to be hospitalised and given lifesaving treatment. Never, ever hesitate to seek medical advice with a red-hot swollen boob. It needs to be nipped in the bud immediately. Trust me, I've had it eight times in total and it's the absolute pits. Or should I say, tits.

Thrush

Hell yeah, you read that right. Not only can your flaps develop into a hot yeasty mess, so can your baps! Oh, and your baby's mouth too! The joy. Symptoms of nipple thrush include itchy, flaky or shiny skin on the areola or nipples. Red or cracked nipples, and stabbing pains within your breasts during or between feedings.

But this is the really fun part; left untreated you and your baby will keep passing that fungal delight back and forth to each other quicker than an STD during Freshers' week. So don't go applying that year-old tube of Canesten you found buried at the back of the cupboard, get yourself to your GP and they'll prescribe treatment. But make sure they prescribe treatment for BOTH of you or the infection will just keep on going and going and going!

Vasospasms

Say what now? I'm including this one because I personally experienced this and at the time I had absolutely no
idea what was happening to my body.

Described scientifically, vasospasm refers to the
sudden contraction of the muscular walls of an artery. It
causes the artery to narrow, reducing the amount of blood
that can flow through it, resulting in stabbing pain, itching and whitening of the flesh where the blood is
restricted. It can happen anywhere in your body but some
women experience it in their nipples while breastfeeding.

How will you know you have them? Well, if feeding
feels like there are two high-voltage electricity currents
shooting out of the end of your nipples, you're probably
suffering from them. You may also notice that your nipple
looks like it has seen a ghost at the end of each feed and
is discoloured or white.

Unfortunately, there's not much you can do about electricity tits, but a poor latch will definitely make it worse.
It's worth seeking professional help for vasospasms, so
contact your GP to discuss or, better still, hire a lactation
consultant.

Breastfeeding grief

Before I move on to share the very positive breastfeeding experience I had with my second child, I wanted to
touch on the concept of breastfeeding grief when your
breastfeeding journey comes to a premature end. By

prematurely I mean before you are mentally and emotionally ready to stop.

Dr Bumfluff helped me to let go of my idealistic view of breastfeeding as the only acceptable way to feed my child, but that didn't lessen the shame or guilt of stopping. It took a couple of days of exclusively pumping to repair my annihilated nipples, but once they were healed I just couldn't face going through the ordeal of breastfeeding again. I attempted a few feeds, and that familiar feeling of having my norks ground through a meat mincer was very much present so I decided to continue pumping and introduce formula.

Over the next few weeks, the pumping lessened and Oliver slowly moved exclusively to formula. I felt such a sense of relief that I didn't have to endure the toe-curling agony of breastfeeding any more. I was much more relaxed and confident in my ability to mother my child, and guess what, we were bonding! Whereas before I would look at him and only see the threat of his savage gummy latch and the damage he was about to inflict on me, I was finally experiencing the maternal love that had been almost absent since his birth. I felt like his mum.

However, that didn't ease the grief of our breastfeeding journey coming to an end. It felt like a loss. We're taught that as women we are biologically designed to feed our babies, yet my anatomy had failed me miserably and it left me feeling bereft. I felt inadequate as a woman, let alone as a mother. It was difficult to shake that feeling and, just like a bereavement, it's taken many years for me to come to terms with it. So if you're reading this, having had a similar experience to me or you're going through the grieving process right now, know that you are not alone and that your feelings are valid. Embrace the grief and mourn, because only by recognising our pain are we capable of moving on. Of course, I have the benefit of hindsight now and having fed my babies in all sorts of ways, I have learnt that how you feed your children is no reflection on your ability to mother them. Tit or teat, either way, kids still end up being little dicks.

Tits at the end of the rainbow

I hope the story of my first breastfeeding experience hasn't left you as traumatised as it left me. I'm pleased to tell you that there is light at the end of this tit tunnel, and although my breastfeeding journey came to an end with Oliver, I did go on to happily combi-feed my daughter two years later.

My first thought when I discovered I was pregnant with her (after, how will my vagina survive another battering?) was whether or not I would breastfeed. My gut reaction was FUCK THAT SHIT, but then once she was here, I decided to give it a go. Armed with the benefit of hindsight and the sweet memory of Dr Bumfluff's cherub-like face, my mindset was completely different and I was adamant that, above all, my sanity would come first.

So I started breastfeeding, but within the first few feeds that familiar sensation of having been attacked by a flesh-eating zombie was compromising my desire to continue. I pumped instead; fed expressed milk, then gave a little formula, attempted another breastfeed and generally mixed it up. I had enough of an understanding of the process of how a milk supply is established that by three weeks in, I was mainly breastfeeding during the day and then pumping/bottle-feeding expressed milk or formula at night. This is known as combi-feeding and it felt bloody fantastic. Now if you've read any literature about breastfeeding, or been to an antenatal class, it's highly unlikely that combi-feeding was discussed. For some reason, it lies outside the norm in the baby feeding world – either you breastfeed or you formula-feed and that's it. Contrary to popular belief, it is possible to successfully combine the two and I am a staunch advocate of the benefits of doing both, not just to Mum, but all the family. Without taking those regular breaks from the tit limpet, giving my body space to heal and also sharing the load of night feeds with my husband, I doubt that I would have continued breastfeeding past those first couple of weeks.

Now if you too decide to go down this route, you need to be prepared for a lot of pumping – and not the sexy kind. I spent many an hour feeling like Daisy the dairy cow with my boobies strapped into an industrial breast pump. Just turning it on and hearing the distinct churning buzz of its motor would get me lactating. I would watch, bemused, at the sight of my nipples being drawn in and out of the flanges like two swollen slugs wearing milk-ejaculating penis helmets trying to escape a polytunnel. Initially I was disheartened by the lack of milk I was producing but I was advised to check out the size of my flange. Excuse me? That's no way to talk about my vagina! Alas, they weren't referring to my cavernous clunge but to the plastic pieces that fit directly over your nipples to form a seal around the areola. Who knew, but the amount of milk extracted is directly linked to the size of your flange. Upon this discovery, hubs excitedly dug out an old WHSmith ruler and we measured my nips together (see, I said it wasn't sexy). THEY WERE F-ING TINY. Pretty unfair given that my areolas by this point were the size of digestive biscuits. But hey, nature is a cunt. Two flange sizes smaller and I was in milky business. I soon adjusted to the ritual of my pumping schedule and as each breast-feed got less painful, I did more titting and less pumping and eventually stopped expressing completely at about three months.

At this point, I really began to relish breastfeeding and for the first time I could understand why women loved it. It was pain-free now, easy, quick, convenient (at times) and I loved the intimacy of feeding my daughter as we lay together, cuddled up snugly skin on skin, in bed. It lived up to my pre-baby breastfeeding fantasies but with the balance of being able to share the responsibility with my husband. It was beautiful.

But just like every other method of feeding, it had its drawbacks. Like the time I ventured out for the day and got stuck on the A406 with a screaming hungry baby. I would normally take a bottle out wherever I went for those 'just in case' moments, but guess who packed the bag that day? Daddy dickhead. What a wanker. So there I was, in the driver's seat heading to see my friend when Edith starts stirring. Oh no. Oh no no no. Her grunts quickly escalated to piercing screams and my body was hit with a rush of anxiety that had my blood pressure soaring and my bumhole twitching. Traffic had come to a standstill, we were miles from our destination and the likelihood that I could stretch my tit all the way to the back seat to feed her was looking low. There was nothing I could do and it didn't take long before hysteria set in. For the both of us. In my panic. I turned on the radio and tuned in to some static in the hope that the white noise might prove calming. It only seemed to rile her and so we spent the next ten, long, horrendous minutes to the next junction hysterically crying to the soundtrack of constant power spectral density. It put me off driving anywhere with her for about six months and reminded me never to let my useless twat of a husband anywhere near the baby bag.

In the end, I combi-fed Edith for almost a year with breastfeeding forming a large proportion of that journey. Unlike the grief I experienced when I stopped breastfeeding with Oliver, this time round our journey ended and all I felt was pride. The biggest lesson that I've learnt is not to let other people's opinions about your feeding choices get in the way of how you want to feed your baby. If truth be told, I think many of our breastfeeding ideals and expectations are dictated by other people's opinions and the idealised perception of motherhood. But in my humble experience, no one route is easy, each comes with its own challenges and difficulties and, you know what, we need to give ourselves a fucking break.

Feed them your way

So I want to remind you, ladies, that however you feed your babies – breast, bottle, combi – you are doing the right thing. Take pride in how you feed your child, goddammit, let's bloody well celebrate it and shout it from the rooftops! It's your body, your baby and you, and only you, know what's right for your family.

And to all those judgmental onlookers out there who have an opinion about women's feeding choices, it's none of your goddamn business. Whether that's a GP, health visitor, Aunty know-it-all, Lucy lactation tits at playgroup – when you see a woman feeding her child, whether in public, or online, please keep your useless and quite frankly damaging opinions to yourself. You have no idea what that mother has been through, so rather than putting her down and making her feel ashamed for one of myriad reasons – breastfeeding in public, or breastfeeding for too long or not breastfeeding for long enough, or feeding her baby formula – just check yourself before opening your mouth and maybe, just maybe, don't be a cunt. It's really not that difficult.

And mamas, keep going you absolute queens, you're doing an amazing job. Stand tall, be proud, tits and teeth, and remember – you've fucking got this.

11

SLEEP

The battle of bedtime

If there's one parental obsession that unites new mums and dads across the globe, it's got to be the matter of sleep. Or rather, a lack thereof. Right now, hundreds of thousands of you are staggering around in the dark, bleary eyed and blotchy faced, having just been woken for the umpteenth time by the cries of a hungry baby, wondering 'will this hell ever end?' You are not alone.

Sleep is undoubtedly at its worst during the fourth trimester (the first twelve weeks), with frequent night wakings, short bursts of sleep and irregular sleeping patterns. Now I know that some smug wanker out there will tell you that their baby was sleeping through the night from birth, but I think your best bet is to rein in your expectations of your newborn's sleep and never speak to that twat again. Not, at least, until hearing those words doesn't make you want to smash their face in out of jealousy and tired rage. The bitter truth is that during the newborn phase you're about as likely to get a full night of uninterrupted sleep as I am to get a fingering from Brad Pitt. We can fantasise about it to our heart's content, but it's never going to happen, babe.

But have no fear! This chapter is here to hold your hand through the first three months of newborn sleep-deprivation hell. It'll help you to understand your newborn baby's sleep needs specifically during the fourth trimester, and give you some simple sleep tools that you can implement with your sproglet from day one. From getting to grips with sleep windows and discovering the soothing powers of white noise, to learning how to create the perfect baby burrito, think of this as your SOS newborn sleep survival guide. Because that's the aim here, people: SURVIVAL.

The science bit

Newborn babies actually sleep a remarkable amount, and in the first few weeks will rack up an average of 11–18 hours of shuteye every day. But despite all this kip, you're still going to develop eyebags that look like the testicles of an eighty-year-old pensioner, as the little pricks will spread it out across 24 hours in bursts of 45 minutes, three hours at a time.

Why this erratic bellendary? Well, babies' stomachs are tiny, so they need to be filled frequently, which means lots of wake-ups for feeding. Plus, unlike you and me, their circadian rhythm has not yet synchronised with the external, 24-hour cycle of daylight and darkness that governs our sleep patterns, meaning they make no distinction between day and night. Erm, WTF is a circadian rhythm? Well, in simple terms, it's your internal body clock telling you the right time to be awake versus asleep. It does this by releasing specific hormones at specific times, to create a stable cycle of restorative rest at night and wakefulness during the day. Pretty much every living organism has one – except your stupid baby.

Is there anything you can do to bring their body clock more in line with yours?! Sure, you can start to encourage their body clock to adapt to the same pattern as yours by ensuring they get plenty of sunlight during the day, and then lowering the lights and keeping things relatively dark in the evening, but in all honesty, you're just going to have to roll with it. It's helpful, however, to know that the constant broken sleep is not down to you doing something wrong, or that you've been cursed with a broken baby. Your kid sleeps like a twat because biology made them that way. Good news is, their circadian rhythm begins to develop at around ten to twelve weeks, when they will naturally begin to sleep for longer stretches at night. At this stage they are also developmentally ready to respond to a bedtime routine, so you can start implementing some structure if you wish to.

Despite the intermittent sleep, it may seem that your newborn is actually asleep more than they're awake (except when you want them to be) but there's good reason for all that slumber. Although they appear to be less active than a sedated slug, the reality is that an enormous amount of physical and mental development happens while they're sleeping. These developments help brain functions mature and influence critical abilities such as language, attention and impulse control. Brain activity during sleep also has a direct effect on a child's ability to learn and may even affect developmental and mood disorders. So they might just seem like lazy buggers but they're actually very busy.

It goes without saying that a baby who gets enough sleep is going to generally be more agreeable, less fussy, easier to soothe and more responsive. You've probably already discovered that most adults are pricks without sleep, well the same applies to babies. However, the massive difference between us and them is that we can self-regulate when we need sleep but babies have not yet developed that ability.

By self-regulation, I mean that we understand and manage our behaviour and our reactions to feelings and things happening around us and respond appropriately. So, if we're tired, we recognise our tiredness and respond by going to bed early. Or if you're like me, just ignore it and stay up to watch one more episode of the box set you're currently bingeing and then regret it massively in the morning. Babies, however, rely on us to manage a large portion of their regulatory needs, from whacking a tit in their mouth when they're hungry, to popping a jumper on them when they're cold, to helping them fall asleep when they need us to. They can react physically to the sensory information around them, but they've got a long way to go before they can take themselves off to bed and fall sleep independently.

So, forget the myth that 'babies will sleep when they are tired.' It's a load of old bollocks. If that were the case, they'd be a hell of a lot fewer knackered parents out there losing their minds trying to get a baby to sleep. It's up to us to help our babies *fall* asleep, figure out *when* they need to sleep and ensure they get *enough* sleep to enable that integral development to happen.

OK, so how the hell do you do all that then? Cue the manifestation of your inner nap ninja. *Hi-yah!* (Insert karate chop here.)

The magic window of sleepy bliss

Your first step to nap ninja enlightenment is to familiarise yourself with your baby's awake window. Excuse me, what now? Awake windows are the periods of time that your baby is awake between each nap and their night-time sleep. Every child, based on their age, has a maximum threshold of time that they are able to stay awake depending on where they are in their development. As babies get older their window of wakefulness gets longer, they'll generally nap for longer, and the number of naps they need will gradually decrease and become more predictable. At 0–3 months old, your baby's awake window is anywhere between 45 and 90 minutes, meaning they'll be having roughly 4–8 periods of sleep a day.

A few newborn babies will just fall asleep no matter what (you lucky bastards) whereas, as we've discovered, the majority of babies are going to need your co-regulatory input to nod off. Some babies will give you very good clues that they are tired (see sleep cues) so you can start soothing as soon as they look a little glazed over. Then there are the babies (bellends) who seem to actively fight sleep and stay awake far longer than they can handle.

At this age, most babies need roughly 16–18 hours of sleep over the 24-hour period, and if they sleep for less than this amount, they are likely to be overtired. You'll know THIS is your baby if they stay awake for 1.5 hours or longer and enter mega overtired meltdown territory. If we can, we want to avoid overtiredness like it's an STD.

So, you've got two objectives here, ninjas:

• Ensure your baby has enough awake time in between naps to build up sleep pressure.
• Make sure you put baby down for sleep before they become overtired.

Simple, right?! As every baby is different, you're going to have to do a bit of nap ninja detective work to determine where your baby's magic sleep spot falls – you'll know you've hit it when baby falls asleep quickly and with little fuss. But if it takes you an age and feels like one massive losing battle (assuming you've eliminated factors like hunger and wind) you're either trying too soon or you're trying too late.

Most of the time it's the latter, and as you will no doubt discover for yourself, an overtired baby is as volatile as an unpinned hand grenade – small, angry and capable of creating mass destruction. Trust me, I've got the injuries to prove it.

Let me give you one such example. Having no concept of these awake windows, we took Oliver off to his cousin's second birthday party when he was just six weeks old. Now if you've never been to a two-year-old's birthday party, I think it would be best described as absolute fucking carnage. It's like hanging around with a bunch of miniature drunks, only these wreck heads are tanked up on adrenaline, Capri Sun and unicorn cake. So, while ten rowdy toddlers ran riot, screaming with excitement and thrashing around the house, Oliver and I sat there, stunned into a silent stupor. It was our first proper outing outside the calm and chilled sanctuary of our house so the noise, the bustle, the fact that a small child kept shouting 'baa baa black sheep' aggressively into our faces – it was quite a sensory over-load.

Overstimulated to the hilt, there was no way this kid was having a nap surrounded by toddler mayhem. By the time we left, he was so wired that even the car jour-ney home didn't send him off. I was scared. It was the longest period of time he had ever been awake; we're talking three hours plus, and I could sense that he wasn't in a good place. Now foolishly, rather than just pull out all my soothing skills and get him to sleep, I decided instead to give him a bath. WHAT WAS I THINKING?

As soon as I'd got him undressed, the crying started and then as I lowered him into the water, it was like I'd unleashed a demon. He screamed a blood-curdling scream and the cries were coming so thick and fast that it literally took his breath away. You would have thought I was trying to murder him, when all I was trying to do was give his balls a little rinse. And the screaming did not stop. We whipped him out of the water and took him to a dark room to try to calm him down, but the crying was relentless. To be honest, he hadn't really cried a huge amount since he was born, so it was a terrifying shock to the system to suddenly be confronted by this red-faced furious baby who was barely inhaling a breath between each ear-splitting scream. We genuinely didn't know what to do with him and pretty soon I was crying as hysterically as him. In our panic, Rob Googled how to stop a baby crying and read that blowing a puff of air into their face helped to calm them down. So, there we were, Rob blowing into Oliver's face, Oliver looking at him as if to say 'what the fuck are you doing?' and me in a heap, rocking back-wards and forwards feeling we'd genuinely broken our baby.

Eventually, with a lot of soothing, we managed to calm him down and get him to sleep, but it was honestly one of the most stressful moments I've ever had as a parent. Probably because it was the first time I ever had to deal with a screaming baby who was out of their mind from overtiredness. So, the moral of the story is this – be mindful of your baby's awake window and do whatever it takes to get them to sleep within it. Sure, it won't always go to plan, you'll have good days and bad days, but generally, sticking to these awake windows does take a lot of the stress out of getting your baby to sleep. Plus, if you're aware of how long your baby has been awake and they slip over the threshold, it won't be such a shock to the system when they start behaving like they've been possessed by the devil. You'll know exactly what's going on and can pull out all your soothing tools to chill them out and hopefully get them to sleep.

The 'good baby' myth dispelled

As a parent, I can guarantee that you will be asked this ridiculous question a million times in the first year of your child's life. 'Is s/he a good baby?' which actually translates to 'does your baby sleep?' Those whose babies are 'good' and do sleep are congratulated. Those whose babies are 'troublesome' and don't sleep, receive sympathy and unsolicited tips on how to improve their sleep habits.

Alongside your feeding choices, it seems sleep is one of the first areas of parenting by which new parents are judged by others. From where your baby sleeps, to how long they sleep, to whether or not they fall asleep independently – everyone has an opinion.

But you know what? Fuck off. Your baby's ability to sleep is not a reflection of their personality being 'good' or 'bad', neither is it a reflection of your ability to parent. It's easy to forget that babies, even when they're in the slug-like newborn phase, have their own temperament. Every single baby is an individual and will have their own unique sleep needs and it's nobody else's business how those manifest. And what works for one baby will be completely pointless for another. It's all just trial and error.

Fact is, some babies will always struggle with sleep from day one, whereas others will have zero issues. Just as we do as adults. There's no such thing as a good baby! So next time a judgmental twat lays this question on you, you have full permission to turn around and punch them in their moronic mouth.

Watch that baby like a hawk

So, you've just learnt how helpful awake windows can be to achieving easy, stress-free naps, but how do you work out where your baby's sweet sleep spot falls within that window? It's not like the sedated slug can communicate verbally or anything, so what physical cues can you look out for that indicate they're getting ready for sleep?

Of course, every baby will present differently, but typically 0–3-month-old babies can show any of the following sleep cues. But, a warning: some of these signs are so subtle they could go unnoticed, so get ready to activate your ninja hawk-eye observation mode!

Cues that your baby needs to go to sleep:

Whining or crying. Er, yeah, babies do that all the fucking time so this one isn't particularly obvious to the undiscerning eye (or rather, ear). But if they're being especially whingy, then you know you're probably close. But if they're full-blown crying, you've probably missed your moment.

Staring blankly into space. I mean, come on. We've established that the slug-like qualities of a newborn baby and staring into space is their default setting. How can you tell the difference? Just look out for extra-vacant sluggy vibes, a glazed-over expression and whether they turn or look away from anything that may be stimulating to them.

Yawning, stretching and rubbing their eyes. Finally, a cue we can all get on board with! There's literally nothing else more universally accepted as a sign for 'get me the fuck to bed' than the old yawn, stretch, eye-rub routine. Some babies may also pull at their ears, clench their fists or arch their backs when they're getting tired, so look out for those too.

Going quiet and still or moving more than usual. Generally, babies don't make a huge amount of noise (except when they're crying, obvs) but if you notice they're markedly quiet coupled with a slowing down of movement, you've probably got yourself a sleepy little grub. On the contrary, your baby might actually move more than usual. So, if their limbs start randomly jolting with more zeal than Mick Jagger's hips, they're probably tired.

It's important to remember that this is not an exhaustive list of sleepy cues, these are just the most common signs of a tired baby. Every child will act differently when tired and it's up to you to observe and learn what their unique sleep cues are. Don't worry, you'll pick it up pretty quickly given they need sleep every bloody 30 seconds, and once you've mastered the perfect ninja hawk stare, here's what to do next.

The womb room

Before we get to the soothing elements of helping your baby get to sleep at home, let's first take a quick look at their sleep set-up. Now a lot of naps in these early days are likely to take place in your arms and on the move, which is absolutely fine and dandy. Babies are pretty portable at this stage, so don't feel you have to be at home for every single nap, but if you are at home and wish to put them down in a room, in a cot, a bassinet or co-sleeping with you, here's what you can do to create the perfect sleep-conducive environment. We're aiming for the most womb-like conditions here, in a bid to make baby feel the same comfort and security they felt in utero. Ninja, it's time to assemble the 'womb room'.

White noise

The womb is not a quiet place, far from it in fact. From the rhythmic pulse of your heartbeat to the whoosh of your blood pumping round your uterus, to the ambient noises travelling through your belly from the outside world, babies are used to lots of noise. Which may explain why playing certain sounds and sshing you baby can have a calming impact and help them to sleep. But whereas I'm partial to the soothing tones of a pan pipe to assist my relaxation, babies haven't yet developed the same refined music taste as moi. In fact, they're pretty basic when it comes to soothing auditory preferences, and most babies are mad for a bit of white noise.

One study of newborn babies found that 80 per cent of those exposed to white noise dozed off within five minutes, while only 25 per cent of those without the background noise fell asleep as quickly. White noise is also thought to improve the quality of baby's sleep, since it contains all frequencies at equal intensity and can mask loud sounds that stimulate their tiny brains, helping them to stay asleep for longer periods of time. Give them the hum of a hairdryer or the whirr of a desk fan and they're buzzing, or should I say, snoozing.

For maximum benefit, start playing the white noise as soon as you begin settling baby and leave it on for the duration of their sleep. As it's neither safe or practical to leave a hairdryer on for a prolonged period of time, your best bet for playing it continuously is via a white-noise machine. You can also play it via YouTube on your phone or tablet or download a white noise app. The only downside to that option is having to sacrifice your phone at every nap time, when we all know you'll want it to scroll aimlessly through Instagram while they sleep to stop you from going out of your mind with the boredom of parenthood.

Blackout

Not only is the womb noisy; it is also dark. As you know, your baby's circadian rhythm is an absolute joke at this early stage, but that doesn't mean they won't benefit from sleeping in a dark room. This is because light suppresses the production of melatonin, which is the hormone that makes us sleepy. As a result, babies fall asleep and stay asleep more easily in a darker room than when there's light beaming in telling their body it's time to be awake. A dark room is in fact a critical aspect of helping baby's sleep, especially with early morning wake-ups, fostering longer naps and maintaining early bedtimes despite it being light outside.

So, what you're aiming for here, is a blacked-out room. Now when I say blacked-out, I mean BLACKED out. You want that room as dark as feasibly possible. As a basic requirement, I'd say you need at least a blackout roller blind plus blackout curtains to achieve the desired darkness level. Personally, I went full nutjob with the blackout situation and fashioned my own homemade blackout system that involved three impenetrable layers of light-banishing material: foil at the window, blackout roller blind, blackout sheet Velcroed to the window frame. I mean, the foil on the windows may have been a tad excessive but when you're that desperate for your baby to sleep, you're even willing to forgo all your interior design goals and embrace the aesthetic of a crack den.

Swaddling

Swaddling is the practice of wrapping your baby up like a human burrito to calm them down and aid restful sleep. See, newborn babies are jerks. Yeah, we know that, but what's swaddling got to do with it? Well, babies jerk off a lot. Do they?! Not in the sense that they fiddle with their bits, but they will frequently jerk themselves awake from sleep due to their incredibly sensitive startle reflex. You'll be witness to this jerk action when your baby suddenly extends their arms and legs, arches their back or quickly curls in like they've just received a surprise poke up the bum. These reflexes aren't intentional, but instead are basic motor responses. So, although it may appear they are auditioning for the role of Beyoncé's backup dancer, they're just reacting to the environment around them.

Swaddling can help prevent unnecessary wakeups caused by the startle reflex by keeping baby's flailing Beyoncé limbs contained. It also has the added benefit of making babies feel snug and secure just like they did in your tummy, thus stimulating prolonged sleep continuity – baby burrito them up and they'll rouse less and sleep for longer.

The practice of swaddling is fairly straightforward and can be achieved in a number of ways, either using a large muslin cloth or purchasing special swaddle blankets/pouches. The easiest way is with the latter, as there's no messing about with excess fabric and ending up with a sloppy burrito that baby can easily escape. Just ensure you are following safe sleep practices (check the Lullaby Trust, www.lullabytrust.org.uk, for expert advice on safer sleep) and research swaddling thoroughly before attempting to swaddle your baby. By three months you want to ensure that your baby no longer needs a swaddle and has their hands out so that they can integrate this reflex and get used to sleeping in a sleeping bag instead.

Soothe that sucker to sleep

Right! So, let's assume that you've seized the opportune moment in your baby's awake window; you're in the dark sanctuary of the womb room, baby is swaddled and the white noise is ringing in your ears. Now what? Will baby just magically fall asleep?

Now, if you've already read a ton of baby sleep books (which I bet you have) then you're probably familiar with the phrase 'put them down sleepy but awake'. Well, I want you to forget that, the aim here is 'get that fucker to sleep'. That goal comes later down the line when your baby is more able to self-regulate and is capable of learning to fall asleep independently. But for now, you'll have to put in the work and pull out all your ninja soothing skills to get baby to sleep. Just to note here, girls, that some kids are naturally better sleepers than others, no matter what you do. Personally, I have one of each, and everything that worked with my first was utter bullshit with my second. That little sleep sabotager has always hated sleep, and continues to do so. What I'm trying to say is, despite your best efforts, sometimes you just have to deal with a crappy sleeper. But it's not you, it's them. So don't beat yourself up about it. But here are some techniques to help your baby nod off.

Rock'n'roll 'em into bed

Babies are movement junkies – rocking, swaying, bouncing, doing cartwheels (OK, not that one), they love a bit of motion to help them nod off. The effects of rocking on sleep are actually tied to rhythmic stimulation of the vestibular system. What the hell is that?! It's the sensory system responsible for receiving information about our bodies in relation to their movement in space, as well as the acceleration and deceleration of movement. Steady, repetitive movement has a hypnotic effect. Which explains why babies can't resist the seductive lull of the car/pushchair/sling. Incredibly, studies have shown that rocking can help babies and adults to fall asleep faster and, once asleep, spend more time in non-rapid eye movement sleep. This means sleeping more deeply and waking up less. Yes please!

There are lots of ways you can use motion to get your little one to sleep; rocking from side to side, swaying up and down, even bouncing is effective. Some babies like a gentle waver while others prefer a forcible swing, so experiment with what works for your baby. Personally, my kids loved a hard sharp squat action and god knows how many hours I spent aggressively squatting a baby to sleep in the dark. I've got exceptionally well-defined glutes to prove it. I thoroughly recommend getting yourself a rocking chair for these early months, as it means you can rock to your thighs' content, plus simultaneously feed if you need to, without breaking your back and your arms falling off. A birthing ball also does the trick.

Once baby has nodded off you can try transferring them to their cot by gently sliding them out of your arms on to the mattress. But a warning – the arm-to-cot transfer is probably one of the most tense experiences you'll ever go through as a parent as there's a high probability baby will wake up, and that the 20 minutes you just spent bouncing like a dickhead will have to be started all over again. It helps to imagine that you're a bomb disposal expert in this moment and make the transfer with the same delicacy and precision you would apply to handling an undetonated bomb. I mean, it's only going one of two ways, right? Sleep or death (or at least wishing you were dead when their eyes ping open and it's back to square one). You can help the transition from arms to cot by warming up their bed with a hot water bottle or warm towel before making the switch.

Baby bongo

If you don't fancy squatting your way to the thigh definition of Usain Bolt, you can try patting your baby to sleep instead. This has the added benefit of baby starting off in the crib, removing the sphincter-twitching stress of the dreaded arm-to-cot transfer.

Just like motion, babies love touch. We all know the benefits of skin-to-skin contact, but applying weighted pressure to our bodies has a similar calming effect. Patting stimulates the proprioceptive system, which is linked to the vestibular system and informs us of our body position in space, which calms and modulates the central nervous system and, in turn, lowers baby's state of arousal. Basically, patting chills them the f out and helps them to fall asleep.

When patting, keep a steady, rhythmic beat and stick to one area of the body. You can pat with one hand or two, whichever takes your fancy. I like to call this two-handed technique 'baby bongo' and would experiment by patting out my favourite songs to see which they responded to best. Hands-down winner was 'Another One Bites the Dust' by Queen. Five minutes of that classic and they couldn't resist sleep! I mean, you're going to spend three months and beyond doing this shit, so you may as well have fun with it.

You can start with a firm pressure and gradually lighten your touch as they drift off and then stop. Or if, like me, you're too much of a scaredy cat to withdraw completely, you can remove the patting element and just rest your hand on their body until you're certain they are asleep ... which FYI could be hours. If there are any inventors out there, please design a weighted baby sleep glove and get yourself on *Dragons' Den*.

Emergency sleep tools

So, I wanted to throw this in here as there will 100 per cent be times when sleep goes down the absolute shitter and your kid just WILL NOT SLEEP. Generally, if the soothing process exceeds 30 minutes and you can see baby is entering dangerous overtired territory, I'd cut your losses and pull out one of the following emergency sleep tools:

The car

Oh, the trusted car nap! Nothing works faster to get those eyelids dropping than a quick spin round the A406. Sure, it's not that environmentally friendly, but I'm willing to sacrifice a tree or two if it means my baby goes to sleep.

The pushchair

Like the car, the pushchair provides the perfect vehicle for a quick induction into sleep with very little effort on your part. Whack them in, set the seat to recline and pound the streets like a lunatic until that dickhead goes to sleep. Not so great when you forgot your anorak in the panic to get out, you're still in your pjs and torrential rain hits.

The sling

Love a good sling nap – especially great when you don't fancy a 3-mile walk in the rain to get them to sleep. You can pop the sling on at home for a nap or when you're out and about. It's especially useful for those coffee catch-ups with your mum mates when you don't want to leave but baby needs a sleep. Extra points if your tit is floppy enough to simultaneously breastfeed while slinging it up. Honestly, it's a game changer that one. Although a bit of a shock for the checkout lady in Home Bargains when we both realised my areola was staring her in the face as I purchased my multipack of family biscuits.

Everybody loves a bosom for a pillow

Breastfed or bottle-fed, all babies relish a milky teat in their gobs, especially when it comes to bedtime. In fact, out of all the soothing techniques, this is probably the most reliable sleep aid in existence. But why is it so effective?

Well, if you're breastfeeding, you'll be providing an abundance of oxytocin through skin-to-skin contact as well as jizzing it out of your tits into their bodies as you feed. As we know, oxytocin has incredible calming properties and will most certainly help to soothe your baby and send them off to sleep. There is also the possibility that breastfeeding in the evening increases a baby's levels of melatonin (the hormone that helps us become drowsy) as you pass some of your own reserves of this sleep-inducing gold through your milk.

But wouldn't that mean bottle-fed babies weren't as easy to feed to sleep? In theory, yes, but in my experience, breast or bottle, it never made a blind bit of difference. So long as milk was being extracted into their mouths, they were happy. A better explanation then might be that feeding to sleep is effective because it is actually linked to sucking and food intake. Both of these actions release oxytocin, which explains why I get an absolute wide-on eating cake. While suckling and feeding, baby will be producing their own source of sleep-inducing oxytocin, leaving them content, relaxed and ready to cop some zzs.

Some babies will still want to suckle long after they've taken their feed. However, it's not realistic or possible to leave your nip or a bottle in your baby's mouth all night, so you can introduce a dummy if you so wish.

Don't be a dummy ... get one!

This leads perfectly into my paragraph of dummy appreciation. Now I have to admit that I was a massive anti-dummy wanker before I had kids. I have no idea where my distaste for it originated but I was staunchly convinced that my babies would never have one. Fast-forward to two weeks into motherhood with nipples like chewed-up salami and a baby who never bloody slept. Against all my misguided, uneducated precon-ceptions, I drove to Asda and bought four of the fuckers out of sheer desperation. Best decision I ever made.

I'm sure a lot of well-meaning dickheads (especially the hardcore breastfeeding crew) will advise against one, but for the love of god, don't listen. The dummy has singlehandedly made my parenting journey 85 per cent less challenging. Not only at bedtime and with sleep but also on the days when my babies whinged so much, I wanted to rip my own ears off and eat them. Dummies are immediately soothing, they are portable, cheap and they prevent your nipples from shrinking like two raisins after having a baby latched on using you as a human dummy throughout the night. Using a dummy when putting your baby down to sleep might also reduce the chance of Sudden Infant Death Syndrome (SIDS). I love them. That's not to say all babies will love them too, but hey, it's worth a shot for the benefits they bring.

'But they'll become addicted! It'll interfere with breastfeeding! You'll never get rid of it!' Do your research, Brenda, and piss off. Ever met a twenty-five-year-old who still uses a dummy? No, of course you haven't. If you want to get rid of the dummy at any stage, you can. It's recommended that dummy usage should be gently withdrawn between 6 and 12 months, to avoid possible longer-term problems associated with dummy use (such as ear infections, delays to speech and language or misalignment of teeth). These prob-lems have not been found below the age of one year so don't stress about the long-term impact of using one when your baby is still a newborn. They'll wean off it eventually, but for now, enjoy the silence!

How to stay sane in the depths of sleep-deprivation hell

Congratulations, you have passed the ninja sleep training with flying colours! Navigating these first few months of sleep deprivation is never a smooth ride. But I hope that this chapter has given you a better understanding of why it's so chaotic alongside some tools to make the journey through it a little less turbulent. As we've already explored in the previous chapters, your emotional and mental wellbeing can unravel pretty quickly when you're surviving on scattered pockets of broken sleep, and it's easy to see how new parents can become unhealthily obsessed with sleep.

This was certainly the case for me. As someone who thrives on structure, I found the unpredictability of my baby's sleep incredibly difficult to cope with. My reaction was to find a solution and try to fix it, but had I been privy to some basic newborn sleep knowledge before having Oliver, my expectations may have been a bit more realistic and I may not have turned into such a controlling nutter.

Unfortunately, sleep deprivation can lead to desperation, especially when you don't fully understand your baby's sleep needs. After reading a lot of shit advice, I started to follow a sleep schedule to the clock rather than following Oliver's individual needs and kept a sleep diary in the hope that I could get him sleeping longer stretches at night. No surprise, it was a disaster.

I mean, I may as well have used the pages of that diary as toilet paper on my shitty anus because they would have been more useful to me. Plus, I would have saved myself the horrific stress of obsessing over sleep to the point of neurosis, while wasting many, many hours of my life trying to force a baby into a strict routine that was doomed to failure from the onset as it worked against his biological capabilities.

It's far more realistic to follow wake windows than a by-the-clock schedule, especially in the first six months of life. So rather than killing yourself trying to establish a structured sleep schedule during this newborn phase, you're better off embracing the sleep chaos and just rolling with the tiny baby fist-sized punches. It's likely that every day will look different, and what works one time won't work the next. But taking a more flexible, easy-going approach (which FYI is against my very nature) will be better for you and for baby. Sleep-training, structure and routine can come later. Everything with kids is just a phase, so this hell won't last forever. Remember, at this early stage the aim is survival, not schedule, your priority should be keeping baby fed and soothed and you'll both be happier. OK, happy is a stretch – but considerably less miserable than I was keeping that completely ridiculous sleep diary.

12

BODY CONFIDENCE

Learning to love your digestive biscuit areolas

Over the course of pregnancy and birth, the female form undergoes a spectacular physical metamorphosis as it is pulled, stretched and distended to epic proportions to accommodate a growing baby. From the bulbous expansion of your belly to the jaw-dropping circumference of your labouring cervix, inside and out, this incredible bodily transformation that occurs to bring new life into the world is nothing short of a miracle. But try telling that to the postpartum bint living with the aftermath of said transformation, with stretch-marked floppy norks hanging to her knees, a nipple beard and a fleshy belly pouch spilling liberally over her maternity leggings eight months after delivery. Chances are, she'll tell you to fuck off and whack you round the face with her newly acquired foot-long tits. You see the thing is, yes, growing and pushing out babies is miraculous, but boy, it doesn't half take its toll on your body.

Now of course we expect our shape and size to change during pregnancy; it's a given! But what about the long-term impact of all that bodily expansion/compression, both externally and internally once the baby has buggered off out your uterus? Should everything just automatically retract back to its pre-baby mass and form, or will there be irreversible and permanent changes to your physicality? For the majority of women, it's likely they will experience the latter, but how those changes present will be dependent on a range of factors – from age, body type and genetics right through to your general health and your lifestyle. And not forgetting that HOW you delivered your baby can also have an impact in the long term – that is, whether you birthed vaginally or had a Caesarean.

Bearing children is a huge physical ordeal, and very few of us escape the experience without acquiring a few additional lumps and bumps, a little extra droop here and there and the occasional release of piss involuntarily escaping our battered pelvic floors. Bodily changes after pregnancy and birth are completely normal and are testament to the incredible journey your body has been on while growing a child. But when we live in a society that has indoctrinated women with impossible and unrealistic beauty standards that revere the 'perfect' body as slim, toned, pert and not a hint of fanny sag, coming to terms with these changes can be challenging. Some women will embrace every inch of their flappy bits unconditionally, but for those of you who have ever struggled with body image and self-confidence issues as I have, self-acceptance may take a bit more work.

That's where this chapter comes in! Not only will I lay out some of the bodily changes you may expect to see but also how we can learn to block out those negative and damaging beauty ideals and truly love and appreciate the wonder that is your body. Whether you end up with deflated fun bags, lopsided labia or a leaky snatch, hopefully you will finish this chapter feeling empowered by your postpartum wobbling bits and truly believing that you are beautiful and worthy just the way you are. Because – news flash – you are!

Bouncing back is bullshit

It feels apt to begin this chapter by exploring the term 'bouncing back' after birth, as it's a phrase that's frequently bandied around (by twats) in relation to women's postpartum bodies. I'm sure you've heard it before, whether it has been directed at you or not, but exclamations of, 'Wow, she bounced right back' or, 'God, it doesn't even look like she's had a baby!' are considered the ultimate compliments to give a new mum. Apparently, returning to your pre-baby shape and size with little sign that you ever went through the process of pregnancy and birth in the first place is some sort of achievement that deserves to be celebrated. Now as harmless as this well-meaning accolade may appear, in my opinion, it does far more damage than good.

By definition, the term relates to overcoming a shitty experience or event, like an illness or a setback, so when it's used in the context of postpartum bodies, it automatically frames the post-pregnancy body as something negative that needs to be 'got over' and left behind. This is in stark contrast to the way the female form is viewed DURING pregnancy, when women are revered as being at their most radiant and beautiful, with the pregnancy 'glow'. But as soon as that kid has shot out of your chuff, it's game over, babe. There's no recognition of the incredible changes your body has undergone or appreciation for the hard work it took to grow and nurture a baby. No. Phrases like 'bouncing back' only serve to perpetuate the idea that post-pregnancy bodies need to 'snap back into shape' and erase all evidence that pregnancy and birth ever even happened in order to be considered beautiful again.

Unfortunately, this is only fuelled by the depiction of postpartum bodies in the media, press and social media, where the only mums who seem to be celebrated publicly are the ones who live up to that expectation. No doubt we're all familiar with the photos of celebs strutting their perfect stuff with sculpted abs and tits up to their eyeballs a few days after giving birth, looking like they've barely expelled a fanny fart let alone a baby. Sure, a handful of women will look like that postpartum, but what about the rest of us bitches? Reality is, the majority of us will be bleeding a tsunami out of our vages, unable to even look at a bikini let alone manage to squeeze our massively swollen vulvas into one. But funnily enough that never makes it on to the cover of *Heat* or *Take a Break*, does it? It's too raw and too real and quite frankly too much for the patriarchy to deal with.

This rhetoric of perfection in relation to the female form is nothing new; women have endured this bullshit for decades. We've been brainwashed to believe that we should strive for perfection and embody normative feminine beauty ideals in order to be considered beautiful and achieve personal and professional success. But guess what? It's just a fucking illusion created to make us feel bad about ourselves so that we buy more shit to lose weight/age less/be attractive and maintain the status quo that a women's only purpose is to look pretty for the benefit of men. Just look at the body types of women we see in advertising, fashion and TV – 99 per cent of them look exactly the same, with no obvious physical flaws or imperfections and, oh yeah, is it any surprise that those industries are also predominantly run by a bunch of penises? It's the patriarchy in action, babes!

Regardless of whether you've forced a human bowling bowl out of your clam or not, you're expected to comply but, come on guys, give us a break! Was getting torn a new arsehole and sacrificing our sphincters to the anal grape gods not enough for you sadistic wankers?! You want us to don a g-string three days after bumhole and vaginal Armageddon and look like a Victoria's Secret model? Well, fuck that, and fuck you!

Whether or not we return to our pre-baby body and the rate at which we do it should not be revered as some form of achievement or upheld as a beauty goal. Every postpartum body is going to present differently and the fact is, most of us won't 'bounce back' in the way that the media leads us to believe we should. It's just a wildly unrealistic expectation. And what are we even supposed to be 'bouncing' back to? A six-pack and nipples that point in the same direction? Never going to happen, love, because here's the thing: I never looked like that PRE birth and frankly I never will. I ain't got the genes, mate, and neither have the majority of the population.

So let's just all fuck off this idea of 'bouncing back' and stop using it as a compliment. It's great if you can slip into size-10 skinny jeans without your camel toe gobbling your gusset, but it's also great if your body looks completely different from how it used to. Let's do women a massive favour and reframe the celebration of postpartum bodies to honour the awesome transformation our bodies undergo through pregnancy and birth, rather than how tight our arses are or how wide our thigh gap is. No matter what your body looks like after kids, it deserves to be honoured. Whether your norks are still pert little baps or they hang like two hotdogs down to your ankles, or whether your stomach is tight and toned or soft and doughy: IT. IS. NOT. A. REFLECTION. OF. YOUR. WORTH. You nurtured a life for nine months, FFS, and then managed to squeeze it out of a hole the size of a Cheerio. Like I said in the opening paragraph of this chapter, your body is nothing short of a miracle, so let's give it the respect it deserves. All postpartum bodies are beautiful. PERIOD.

Things that helped to nurture my body confidence

Shaking my ass

One of the most powerful tools I use to manage my self-esteem, anxiety and body confidence issues is exercise. It's always been a part of my life but since having kids the focus has shifted from exercising to be thin, to exercising to feel strong. You don't need to be aiming for a six-pack here, we just want to feel that our bodies can carry the weight of motherhood – physically and meta-phorically.

Of course, there are physical benefits to exercising, but it's the neurological benefits that have the biggest clout when it comes to improving your overall wellbeing. Exercise improves cognitive functioning, mental health and memory and helps to:

- Decrease stress
- Decrease social anxiety
- Improve processing of emotions
- Prevent neurological conditions
- Leave you feeling euphoric (in the short term)
- Increase energy, focus and attention
- Hinder the ageing process
- Improve memory
- Improve blood circulation
- Decrease 'brain fog'

I mean, hello! If ever you needed an excuse to get a sweaty clam, this is surely it. And you don't have to be partaking in intensive HIIT workouts to reap the benefits. Just getting your ass off the sofa and moving your body for a daily walk can help. So don't delay, my friend, dig out your Lycra and shake that booty.

Ditch your old clothes if they no longer fit you

Nothing makes you feel like a lump of globus lard like trying to squeeze your postpartum arse into a pair of your pre-baby skinny jeans. Don't do it to yourself, babe. Keep those pre-baby clothes in storage until at least six months after giving birth. And if they don't fit you then, please don't feel bad. They're just clothes and your dress size is not a reflection of your worth. Just don't hold on to them thinking 'one day I'll get back into these and be happy' because that mentally is toxic. Sling them down the charity shop and be free!

Buy something that fits you now

Well, what the fuck am I going to wear now, dickhead? I hear you say. So once you've ditched your old clobber – get yourself some new threads! I've done this after both pregnancies and it's made such a difference to feeling good in my own skin. You don't have to spend a fortune, pick up some staples from the high street or rummage around the second-hand shops, but find a few pieces that bring you joy, make you feel that you look good and, most importantly, FIT YOU! Amazing what a well-fitting pair of jeans can do for your self-esteem. Just avoid anything marketed specifically for mums as that will invariably make you feel like a fusty old hag. Sure, you've got a kid, but you can still be fucking stylish!

Release some serotonin

When the negativity hits me and I'm feeling low, I try to indulge in a few simple activities that boost serotonin production and bring a little relief from my overactive, self-critical mind. In order of my personal preference:

Have a boogie. Studies have shown that music and movement combined elevate dopamine and endorphins, two neurotransmitters responsible for feelings of pleasure and happiness. Dancing also promotes the experience of 'flow', which is an almost meditative state that allows you to focus solely on movement, music and rhythm instead of worries and stresses like 'does my arse look big in this?'. So get in that kitchen, whack on Beyoncé and twerk away your insecurities.

Have a wank. As someone who works from home alone, I wank A LOT. I mean, why the hell not? It makes me feel more connected and in tune with my body, releases a dick load of endorphins, reduces stress, promotes better sleep and unlike sex with my partner, there's no lying in a cold wet patch for hours afterwards. Win-win.

Stare at your baby. Research has shown that the sight of your baby cues your brain to release dopamine, one of the feel-good chemicals in our brains that promotes a sense of happiness. But it only works if it's your baby, so no gawking at a random kid in Tesco.

Indulge in some hippy shit

Remember our affirmations from the hypnobirthing days of pregnancy and labour? Well, indulge in some of that positive mindset action now too, to boost your self-esteem. If you're frequently finding yourself getting caught up in negative self-talk about your body, positive affirmations can be used to combat these often subconscious patterns and replace them with more adaptive narratives. So instead of our internal monologue saying, 'you worthless cunt', you're going to teach it to say 'you are beautiful and worthy.' There's always an element of feeling like a twat when you start on the affirmation journey, but trust me, you tell yourself you are beautiful enough times and you will start to believe it.

Look for body confidence and self-acceptance role models

I do feel that social media has a lot to answer for when it comes to us feeling shit about ourselves postpartum. Let's face it, seeing other mums living a seemingly perfect life and looking like supermodels 24/7 doesn't do much for our self-esteem when we're still in our dirty pjs with egg down our front and a fanny stinking like a farmyard while sitting in a messy house. Please, please, please, never believe everything you see on social media. It's a fucking illusion. No one is perfect. So don't go comparing yourself to others because you're only ever being shown a tiny, cherry picked, highly edited, glossy slice of someone's life. Personally, I say unfollow anyone who makes you feel shit and seek out the accounts that make you feel good about yourself. There's a huge body positivity movement out there and so many incredible role models paving the way to make women of all shapes and sizes realise their beauty. You can search hashtags such as #bodypositivity-movement or #bodypositivity to find them. Surrounding yourself with a body positive community and seeing women who look like you as opposed to an airbrushed Barbie doll really does put things into perspective.

Get your post-baby jiggle on

Now that we've got that cerebral jizz out of the way and established that the patriarchy and their oppressive beauty standards can fucking do one, let's get down to the practical stuff and explore some of the changes you might expect to see in your postpartum body. Like I said previously, every woman will look different after giving birth, but there seem to be some common physical denominators that bring us flappy titted slags together. Here are some of my personal faves that have, for me at least, lingered way beyond the postpartum period.

Jelly belly

Possibly the most obvious and dramatic change to a woman's anatomy during pregnancy is the colossal expansion of her stomach as it stretches out to house a growing baby. Regardless of physicality, whether you're slight, muscular or curvy, it's near impossible to escape pregnancy without gaining some degree of additional belly beef. But once the baby has vacated your uterus and your womb is no longer occupied, what happens to all that extra gut girth? Will your balloon of a belly just shrink back, unaffected by all that inflation, or will you be left with a permanent kangaroo-style fleshy belly pocket attached to your abdomen?

As discussed in the aftermath chapter, your belly may retain its pregnant bulk for a number of weeks after giving birth, then slowly deflate back down to less bulbous proportions as your uterus shrinks to its former capacity. But since the abdominal skin has been stretched and pulled, the reality is, it may never be as taut or plank-like as it once was. Whether it's stretch marks, weakened abs, C-section scarring or a bit of extra flab, most of us will bear some evidence that our bellies spent nine months swelling up like a gigantic testicle.

Despite being naturally fairly slim and living a relatively balanced and healthy lifestyle (bar my weekly Friday night binge of Pinot Grigio and chocolate), this has certainly been my experience. Two years postpartum and my stomach bears all the signs of its former inflation. The silvery streaks of stretch marks, the core strength of a piece of wet spaghetti and the meaty jiggle of a jelly belly. I got it all, baby! But my most notable belly features post-bambinos are as follows:

A belly button with the circumference of the moon. No joke, my vacuous pit could be rented out as an Olympic-sized swimming pool to ants. It's huge, if I wanted to fist it I could (and have).

The stomach wrinkles of a Sphynx cat. You know that weird, creepy looking, bald cat creature that has more skin than skeleton? Yeah, that's my belly. And if I squeeze it all towards my gigantic belly button, said button crater inverts, bringing the additional skin with it to create a sort of geriatric-looking puckered anus. It's my go-to party trick. Seems my stomach epidermis never got the memo to retract, so now I'm left with enough skin to fashion a small parachute. Handy if I ever find myself accidentally thrown out of a plane, but not so great for my self-esteem or for skinny jeans.

The formation of a 'gunt'. Whereas my gut once existed within its own clear and distinct territory, it has now formed a fleshy homogenous alliance with my cunt. The two areas are no longer defined separately and instead haunt me together as one singular mound of gunty blubber. It's the ultimate dynamic duo.

Chipolata underboobs

Now I'm not sure if this is to do with pregnancy or gluttony, but since kids, I've developed two ample sausages of flab that nestle snugly under my tits. I don't know how they got there or what purpose they serve other than creating a permanent clammy nook for my nork sweat to pool into and fester. And it doesn't matter how many sit-ups I do or how many kale salads I eat, my secondary pair of chesticles are here to stay. May as well accept it and start double bra-ing those fuckers.

Foot-long hairy hotdog baps

Have you ever heard of the pencil test? Well, apparently, if you want to gauge how taut your titties are, just take a pencil and place it under your bare boob. If it drops to the floor, congratulations, you have an excellently pert rack. However, if your pendulum-like booby flaps grab on to said pencil and engulf it whole into the vortex of your floppy, foot-long hotdogs, commiserations, you've probably had kids. Fuck the pencil, girls, I can get a bottle of Pinot Grigio under each tit! Welcome to the saggy nork club, mums!

Technically, pregnancy is to blame for this delightful rack sag, due to the changes that occur in muscle structure and function as your body prepares to feed a baby. Your breasts are made up of glands, fat and fibrous tissue and when pregnancy hormones ramp up, extra blood volume causes the tissue to swell, and the glands begin to fill up with breast milk. All of this fluid gain can cause mega-boob syndrome and your breasts become heavy and dense (hello Jordan-esque FF bazookas). Unfortunately, it can also do an absolute number on the connective and fatty tissues (cue tits like tennis balls in sports socks), leaving them looser and thinner, which can affect breast shape and texture in the long term. Yeah, no shit, mate.

But as with everything else relating to pregnancy and birth, exactly how or even if it will change your jubblies is based on your genetics, age, body composition and previous pregnancies. And you won't really know until you're well and truly done and dusted with pregnancy and breastfeeding. Some postpartum bints will have breasts that snap back to pre-baby size (I hate you), or they'll permanently gain a cup size, or even lose a cup size and some women find that their norks are uneven, with one tit noticeably bigger/smaller than the other. And then some unfortunate bitches, like me, will be left with what can only be described as a pair of windsocks on a breezeless day dangling from their chests like two rags, forlorn and lifeless.

I have to admit that of the many changes to my body since spawning my offspring, I mourn the departure of my once-perky norks the most. Gone are the pert, plump pillows of my youth, and instead what I've essentially been left with are two enormous dehydrated skin tags for tits. Taking my bra off is like unfurling a pair of King Charles spaniel ears and, guess what, they are also that hairy. Thanks to those wanker pregnancy hormones messing with my follicles, I now need to groom my canine appendages on a weekly basis. Forget about stray hairs randomly growing out of your chin ladies, it's the areola beard twins you need to worry about. They're only a couple of hairs away from opening up their own artisan coffee shop, popping on a flat cap and serving overpriced lattes in jam jars.

And nipple hair hasn't been the only areola injustice that I've suffered at the hands of my children. Remember the digestive biscuits nips I described in the pregnancy chapter? The gargantuan scale, the drastic colour change, the fact they were so prominent you could see them from space, etc? Well, McVitie nips hung around for quite some time post-birth – almost a year, in fact. But there's hope! Don't be disheartened by possessing enough areola circumference to serve a small buffet on, slowly but surely the biscuit nips should start to shrink back. It took a while but gradually they returned to their pre-baby appearance and are now more akin to a Jammy Dodger than a digestive. I mean, they do face in two completely different directions and grow a whopping four inches when erect, like tiny little penises in my bra, but silver linings and all that.

Pissy fanny hammock

Of all the physical changes your body undergoes due to pregnancy and birth, ending up with a leaky piss hole feels like the biggest kick to your postpartum vag. Floppy windsock tits and a gunt overhang I can accept, but soggy knickers that smell like a public toilet on the regs? NO THANKS!

Unsurprisingly, supporting a human watermelon for nine months subjects your pelvic floor to substantial strain, not to mention the battering it then takes while squeezing out said watermelon. All that pressure can weaken the muscles around your bladder and pelvis, leading to pelvic floor problems including loss of bladder and/or bowel control, pelvic organ prolapse and reduced sensation or satisfaction during sex. Most commonly, pelvic floor issues manifest as either involuntary expulsions of wee being shot out of your flaps when the pelvic floor experiences any tension – i.e. with a sneeze, cough, raucous laugh or sudden movement. Or you may find that the urgency to wee is suddenly very intense and has to be acted upon IMMEDIATELY, or else you end up standing in a pool of your own piss in the middle of Sainsbury's (yes, that happened).

If you find yourself mopping up a damp clam after giving birth, you won't be alone. In the three months after childbirth, it's estimated that half of women experience labia leakage with some cases of the piss pants lasting up to a year. And a smaller percentage of women will still be living with symptoms after five years and beyond.

I too experienced the torment of a torrential twat. During the first few months after my son's birth, I was more likely to be rolling in a wet patch after a sneeze than I was from a rendezvous with my husband. Her royal urineness was a frequent visitor to my pantie palace and we have shared many a magical moment together. Her first and most spectacular entrance took place just three months after said son was born, and it took me by such surprise that I was literally rendered knickerless.

Flashback to a school sports hall on a cold December night, with an unsuspecting moi about to mount a mini trampoline for my first postpartum disco-bounce work-out. The lights went down, the strobe came on and I nervously took my place amongst the rows of Lycra-clad women unsure of what I'd just let myself in for. With the music pumping loudly and the enthusiastic instructor bellowing commands at us like an army general; 'SQUAT', 'LEG RAISE', 'JUMPING JACKS' I launched in with gusto, legs akimbo and arms flapping, propelling myself as high as I could on the trampoline. Suddenly, in mid-air I felt an uncontrollable gush of weighty warmth exiting my pee hole. Horrified that I may have just emptied my entire bladder into the crotch of my leggings but still in the throes of the work-out, I had to establish whether I'd wet myself or deposited a particularly watery deposit of discharge.

It was too dark to see but a quick surreptitious scratch and sniff of the offending area confirmed that, yes, it was a whole lot of wee. Filled with embarrassment, I ran to the loo to assess the damage and was confronted with soaking wet undercrackers that had seeped piss right through my leggings. I desperately wanted to crawl up my own arsehole and disappear for eternity but I'd left my coat with my keys and phone in the hall so had no choice but to return. So I did what every person would do in these circumstances – gave my minge a quick blast under the hand dryer and utilised my best *Blue Peter* skills to fashion a panty liner out of a handful of toilet paper to stuff down my knickers.

Back to the trampoline and I carried on jumping, but almost immediately felt my makeshift piss-catcher dislodge just as a second wave of pissnami hit my keks. Filled with panic but in the throes of jumping squats, I tried to stop it slipping any further down my leg, but gravity was against me and the force of each jump pushed the scrunched-up rag of shame further and further down my leggings as my crotch grew wetter. Thigh, knee, calf and then, HELLO! My homemade piss rag finally exited by my ankle and made its dirty escape on to the trampoline between my feet where it lay illuminated brightly in the UV light and continued to unravel in perfect time to the beat of Beyoncé's 'Single Ladies'.

Luckily, no one seemed to notice my pissy drama unfolding during that exercise class and at the end of the session I confided in the lovely instructor, who very sweetly reassured me that it happened frequently to the ladies taking part. It was certainly an experience that I'll never forget, but the biggest lesson I took from it (aside from the tip I was given to always wear patterned leggings when exercising) is how important our pelvic floor health is to both our physical and mental wellbeing. It may not seem obvious but possessing an uncontrollable gushing gusset can deeply impact on our body confidence and our sense of worth.

There's still a lot of shame and embarrassment around urinary incontinence, with many women choosing to suffer in silence rather than seeking professional help, believing that it's a given that you piss yourself post kids. Well, it doesn't have to be that way! Sure, urinary incontinence is a common problem, especially in relation to childbirth, but there's a difference between it being common and 'normal'.

It is not normal to continue experiencing a leaky snatch in the long term after giving birth, so if you find yourself frequently dealing with a dribbly fangita, address it and seek help when it's needed. Goes without saying that pelvic floor exercises are an absolute must for your recovery, so make sure you're doing them right (see the pregnancy chapter for instructions), invest in a pelvic floor trainer (I recommend the Elvie pelvic floor trainer) and seek medical guidance from your GP or a pelvic floor specialist if it's impacting on your day-to-day life. You deserve to feel confident in your body and to jump on a trampoline without the fear of a piss tsunami spontaneously cascading out your vag, so don't just accept it, address it.

Prolonged issues in the lady garden

Very few women get off scot-free from the brutality of giving birth, and for the majority of us, our vaginas will change in one way or another. For some women, there is a small possibility of prolonged complications in the vaginal area that could impact on your day-to-day life and sex if left untreated. The most common issues postpartum are vaginal or anal prolapse, sustained pain during intercourse and urinary incontinence. All of these issues require gynaecological intervention, so don't hesitate to seek medical help if you experience any prolonged complications.

How to find self-love when you feel like a sack of King Edward potatoes

So that's me and my Luna belly-buttoned, wrinkled cat's anus, quadruple-norked midriff, saggy hotdog-titted, leaky hydrant vagina self. There's no flat stomach, no ab definition and most definitely no six-pack (unless six stomach rolls count). Doing a jumping jack without my bra on results in two black eyes from my droopy beanbags punching me in the face and I'm still susceptible to the odd bit of wee escaping my hole now and then.

It's not always comfortable for me to see the physical changes I've undergone having grown two kids – things are bigger, wider, saggier, not to mention much looser. I still occasionally catch a glimpse of my naked body in the mirror, and for that brief moment, I hate what I see. The tits like windsocks, the jiggle of flab, the silvery stretch marks streaked across my body and a huge hairy minge to boot. My inner critic pipes up, 'you should be ashamed of yourself, you look awful, you need to go on a diet, do some exercise you lazy cow, you're worthless.'

Self-loathing will never stop burning, but you know what? I'm done. I'm not listening to that bullshit any more. I've wasted my entire adult life wishing I was thinner, more toned, less wobbly, denying myself food, obsessing over what I eat and, quite frankly, being a miserable cunt because I just wanted a goddamn cheese sandwich. Yes, it makes me feel momentarily inferior that I don't look like my twenty-two-year-old self any more, but I wouldn't want to be her again. I was so unhappy in myself and so hungry. Truth is, I love cake and wine and Brie, and without giving those things up and committing to a gruelling diet/exercise regime or undergoing drastic plastic surgery, this is the way my body looks now and I'm learning to alter my mindset to find peace with that. So I try to be kind to myself, practise body acceptance and remind myself frequently that my body achieved something wonderful and deserves to be celebrated.

My own mother has also unknowingly played a big role in helping me to accept the changes to my body. Having popped out four kids, Mum is no stranger to a stretch mark and, like me, has norks down to her knees and bears the distinct wobble of a postpartum tum. Growing up, I was obsessed with her stomach and loved nothing more than pulling up her jumper and burying my hands (and quite often my face) deep into the silky softness of her midriff. The texture, the consistency, even the smell – it was like kneading a luxurious dough. I'm sure my mum will be delighted that I've just compared her belly to a ball of yeasty flour, but those moments of intimacy with her, stroking her stomach and fondling the space that I had once occupied, filled my five-year-old self with such admiration and pride. To her, it was unsightly and unattractive, but to me it represented comfort and security and connected us in a tangible and visceral way that nothing else did. Well, that's a bit bloody deep but it's true. I don't get to manhandle it the way I used to (because that would be fucking weird), but whenever I'm giving myself a hard time I conjure up the feelings I had caressing Mum's ciabatta loaf. It doesn't matter if my stomach resembles a blancmange, or that my gunt spills over every pair of trousers I own – my body housed my babies, kept them safe, and will forever be a reminder of our journey together bringing them into the world.

We shouldn't be hiding away feeling ashamed and inadequate because we don't fulfil a body ideal projected on us by society; we should be celebrating our gunty beauty and appreciating it for everything it has done for us and our babies.

So you know what I do now when I'm hating myself? I take a deep breath, look straight back at my gigantic minge and give myself a little love. My body is beautiful, I am worthy and the patriarchy can go fuck itself. I urge you to try it for yourself. It's liberating. So let this be a reminder to you to give yourself some appreciation today and every day! We are not defined by the way that we look or by the pounds that we weigh. Let's stop wasting our lives striving pointlessly for an unattainable image of perfection. It's fucking exhausting. Eat the sandwich. Ditch the scales. And dance like your vagina is on fire.

Be kind to yourself, you queens.

13

POST-NATAL SEX

Bracing your blubbery blowhole for impact

And so this brings us right back round to the very sordid act that got us all into this mess in the first place. SEXY TIME, BABY! What's that? I hear you cry. It sounds disgusting. Come on, dig deep, you slag! You remember the days, you know, back when life was full of fun and spontaneity and you did crazy things like going on dates and stayed up past 9p.m. doing shots and getting fingered. And when you woke up with a headache and a sore vagina, it was due to a hangover and too much sex as opposed to an infection in your stitches. Jog any memories? Or what about before you sacrificed your rack to feed a baby and your once-pert coconuts could be caressed and teased without involuntarily spurting lactose? And finally, although this may be particularly challenging to imagine right now, think back to when you harboured a burning desire for your partner and wanted to shag their brains out rather than just wanting to shank them for being such an annoying dickhead.

No? Me neither! And I'm four years postpartum, babe! Being a new parent is all-consuming, and between your leaky tits, the horror of sleep deprivation and the realisation that your partner is a twat, it's no surprise that your sex life can take a bit of a back seat after the birth of your baby.

As we've established, life with a newborn can be immensely demanding, both physically and mentally, leaving you with little time or energy to focus on much else beyond the baby. But there is hope! At some point, when your vagina stops feeling like a punched lasagne and you can safely cough without fear of dislodging an organ or pissing yourself, the odds are, you and your partner will want to resume some semblance of a sex life. So, when do you venture back into the world of willy? How the f do you find the energy to nurture a mutually satisfying sex life with your partner when you haven't had a full night's undisturbed sleep in 230 consecutive days? And probably most pressingly, will sex ever feel the same again with a vagina that's been stretched out like a marquee at a wedding?

Well, the good news is that, yes, of course you can find the fun in your fanny again! Becoming a parent doesn't automatically render you a sexless old crow, it just temporarily messes with your e-QUIM-librium. See what I did there? This chapter will explore some of the barriers that may prevent you from wanting to ride the D, how the dynamics of your relationship may change after having kids and what you can do as a couple to regain a sense of connection and closeness that will hopefully reignite the flames of lust in your knackered loins. Good sex post kids is 100 per cent achievable, so even though your fanny may feel drier than the Sahara Desert right now, with the right communication, some time and effort, plus a whole lot of lube, you'll be slipping and a sliding on that schlong in no time. Let's talk about sex, baby!

Breaking the seal (but hopefully not your stitches)

So let's start with your first foray back into sex after having a baby. When can you expect to bury the weasel after birth? A week? A month? Ten years? Well, the medical guidance states that you should wait six weeks post-delivery before welcoming a sausage into your folds; any earlier than this and your partner may pull out to find your uterus draped forlornly around the end of his dingdong. OK, so that probably won't happen but some couples do genuinely get the mega horn after birth, so much so that they consummate their lust there and then in the delivery suite. No, I'm not joking! Ask any midwife and she'll tell you that's she's walked in to find at least one couple balls deep in fresh post-partum minge. Maybe I'm a prude, or maybe because labour left my flaps feeling like two tattered rags dangling between my legs, but personally, I could not imagine anything worse than getting a porking with my vagina still flapping about like an empty bin bag. Medical guidance is there for a reason, so take it and abstain from vaginal penetration in the first six weeks to avoid causing any further damage to your already pummelled puss and to prevent infection.

Of course, our libidos vary wildly, and for all you know, you may well turn out to be that sex-hungry nymphomaniac getting boned minutes after delivery. Or, like me, you'll be staring at your mangled minge in horror and contemplating committing to a life of celibacy. Either way, desperate to get poked or vowing to never touch another penis again, there's no right or wrong way to feel in this scenario.

Everyone's sex drive is unique, and there are a whole host of factors that can impact on whether or not you want to get jiggy with your partner straight away. You may have had a traumatic birth, your recovery may be slow and difficult, or you may just find the whole experience of becoming a mother so overwhelming and exhausting that you can barely find your feet, let alone find the energy to titillate your clitoris. And let's not forget, this is probably the first time in your life that another human has demanded so much of you on a physical level – whether breastfeeding or not. Come the end of each day, the last thing you want is another body rubbing up against you.

Deciding when you feel ready to be sexually intimate again is going to be a completely individual decision dependent on your experiences of birth, new parenthood and your general physical, mental and emotional wellbeing. For some couples, pum-pum fun may recommence in a matter of weeks, while for others, it could take significantly longer. One study showed that amongst a random group of first-time parents, 14 per cent of the couples had boned within a month, 43 per cent within two months, and 89 per cent waited four to six months before even going anywhere remotely near each other's genitals. I waited three months after the birth of my son and just over a year with my daughter. Perhaps it took us longer the second time round as, with two small children to care for, I barely had the energy to expel a fanny fart let alone snuffle a sausage up my snatch.

Looking back, I realise that I put far more pressure on myself to 'get back to normal' after my son was born and felt that not resuming our sex life immediately was somehow my failing. I've since learnt that 'normal' doesn't exist and the idea that we should all be frothing at the clunge for dick immediately after birth is just another societal construct made up to make women feel bad about themselves. So don't be a mug and fall for it like I did. The important thing is finding what is right for you. Fuck everyone else. Every couple is different, and just because Sally from your NCT group is getting banged three weeks after giving birth, it doesn't mean you have to be too. Remember, what's right for her isn't necessarily right for you and the amount of sex you have or don't have during these first few months of becoming a parent, and indeed at any stage of life, is not a negative reflection of your relationship. And she sounds like a right nobber anyway – personally I'd delete her from the WhatsApp group. Joke! Block her immediately.

Obviously, communication with your partner during this time about how you are feeling and your desire/ lack thereof is key to feeling supported wherever you stand. Of course, your partner will still have their own desires just as you do, but hopefully they are understanding and respectful of how you feel. I mean they bloody well should be, after all, they aren't the one who had to squeeze a human being out a hole the size of a Cheerio. If they put any pressure on you to have sex or deliberately make you feel guilty for not feeling ready, tell the selfish cunt to fuck off and have a wank if they're that desperate. Rob spent twelve months secretly tossing off in the shower after I'd had Edith and it did him absolutely no harm. Sure, he's since developed carpal tunnel syndrome from the repetitive strain injury to his wrists, but we've all had to make sacrifices becoming parents.

Common barriers to boning and how to overCUM them

Feeling self-conscious about your body

The previous chapter was dedicated entirely to body confidence after having a baby, and everything we covered there is also going to apply in the bedroom. Sure, your tits might hang down to your ankles like hotdogs and, yeah, your stomach wobbles like a plate of jelly, but do you know what is really sexy? It's not how many abs you have or how wide your thigh gap is, it's your state of mind. Believe that you are beautiful and sexy – because you are! And if being starkers in front of your partner feels too much, keep the lights low or put on some sexy underwear. It'll make a welcome change from wearing a milk-stained, cottage-cheese-honking nursing bra.

Too tired for tits

Parenthood is exhausting. Period. You will always feel tired, you will always need an early night and your eyebags will always resemble two dehydrated testicles on your face. I'm afraid I don't have a magic solution to fill you with vitality and zest. Just drink bucket loads of espresso, grab every opportunity to nap when you can, never stay up past 9p.m. and occasionally you might just muster the energy to sit on a cock. Although I can't guarantee that you won't then fall asleep mid cunnilingus.

Touched out

Your baby is going to be on you A LOT in the first few months of their life, and you know what, all that physical contact is a lot to process. You may find that by the end of the day you feel totally touched out and the last thing you want is a pair of wandering hands over your body. When you get to this point, try to carve out some time alone away from everyone to reset your brain and your senses. Even if it's ten minutes hiding in a cupboard eating chocolate biscuits, time alone is as integral to maintaining a healthy relationship as spending time together.

Low libido

It's completely normal for both women's and men's libido to hit a rock-bottom low during the first 6–9 months following the birth of a baby. We know that lower levels of oestrogen affect a women's desire for the dong, but studies have shown that men's testosterone levels also dip when they become fathers, leading to a mutual indifference to vajayjay. It's nature's way of preventing another pregnancy! Give yourselves a few months to let your hormones rebalance and you'll be back to rutting like rabbits in no time. And if you aren't at it like you used to be, does it matter? The focus should be on quality over quantity. One magnificently mind-blowing orgasmic session once a month beats three unsatisfactory fumbles a week.

Breastfeeding

This may not seem like an obvious barrier to boning, but having an infant permanently attached to your tits can be a bit of a mood killer. Your breasts' sole purpose now is feeding a baby, and when you're so used to whipping your udders out to nurse, it almost feels a bit odd when you get them out in a sexual context – especially if a tongue is involved. Maybe you fancy a suckling from your partner, but for me, any mouth-to-nipple action was a step too far. If you share this sentiment, make sure you communicate this to your partner and ask them to avoid too much stimulation in the digestive biscuit department. And even without nip play, don't be surprised if your norks are set off during sex and you end up with more than one damp patch. It's just the oxytocin release from having your bits tantalised setting off your letdown reflex.

Let's go to poundtown, baby!

So let's fast-forward and assume that you've reached a place of physical and emotional equanimity. Your beaver is blazing, you're hungry for dick and your pussy is poised, ready for action. Whether this moment arrives weeks or months after delivery, I think it's safe to say that despite the excitement, most women will harbour some apprehension about how this first sexual venture will unfold. I mean, it's not like you haven't tamed the one-eyed trouser snake before, you were like the Pied Piper of penis back in the day, but somehow, taking the initial clunge plunge after giving birth can feel, well, a little intimidating.

So why the worry when you used to happily gobble dick for breakfast? Well, there are myriad factors that may influence how confident you feel getting back into the bedroom. From feeling self-conscious about your postpartum bod and harbouring the fear that you now own a bucket vagina, to the basic logistics of getting jiggy with a baby in the house, through to what you actually do when you come face to penis with your partner for that first time. But don't panic! I'm here to quell your quim qualms and put your mind at rest with my sensual-yet-surprisingly practical guide to getting down and dirty for the first time after giving birth.

So let's address the first issue that came to my mind as I teetered on the cusp of a cunny caress. What exactly is going on 'down there'?

Bucket for a vag

For all you mamas who had a baby plough through their labia and got torn a new arsehole giving birth, I know what you're thinking right now: WHAT IF MY PUSSY FEELS LIKE A FUCKING SUITCASE? I'm with you, babe, you're not alone. In fact, having a cavernous clunge was my biggest worry about having sex again for the first time – quite literally. I knew birth had roughed it up a bit, but my concern was whether or not I'd sustained a permanent fanny expansion. Was it a few extra millimetres I'd gained or was I now harbouring a whale-like vagina that had the square meterage of Heathrow Terminal 4? And if my fanny was indeed now the depth and breadth of a Welsh valley, would sex feel the same way as it had pre-birth? Or would my husband's hotdog be ping-ponging round my walls like a boomerang?

But here's the thing, the human body has incredible healing powers and despite having been brutalised by eight pounds of human flesh, most vaginas do typically return to their pre-baby size a few months after birth, although they may be slightly looser than they once were. This is perfectly normal and how much snatch slack you end up with will be dependent on how much your muscles were stretched during birth and the extent of any tearing (or if you had an episiotomy). Even if you had a C-section, you may experience vaginal weakness after birth, so it goes without saying that practising your pelvic floor exercises regularly is essential for all women post-delivery. It's a muscle, remember, and the more you work it, the stronger and more toned it will become. And if a taut twat wasn't incentive enough, strengthening it also leads to longer, more intense orgasms – and who doesn't love those?

So what does this mean for your love-making experience? Does a wider berth have an impact on your enjoyment of sex? Well, it really depends on the individual and how birth has affected you physiologically, but the extra girth may make it more challenging to achieve an orgasm from penetration alone. It is also common to experience some pain during this first penile encounter, and indeed thereafter for the first six months after birth. Again, this is down to any vaginal changes that have been brought about by birth, and increased sensitivity around scar tissue if you had any tears or stitches. You can minimise the minge ache by using lube, taking it slow and experimenting with positions – all of which I go into further detail about later on in this chapter.

My first tentative step into sex after birth certainly reflects this experience. Having gone without any pum-pum action for months and months on end, it was a massive shock to my anatomy to suddenly be dealing with a foreign object thrusting in and out of my flaps. The labia alarm bells were ringing loudly and I couldn't help but panic that my perineum was going to re-bust open all over my husband's penis. Thank god it didn't, and with each pump, the fear lessened and I started to relax, and hey, I'd even say I started to enjoy it. And despite my genuine concern about having a massive flange, my fears were unfounded. As my husband lovingly exclaimed after he'd shot his load into the abyss of my cervix 'it felt exactly the same'. And who said romance was dead?

So there you go, birthing a child doesn't automatically ruin your vagina. Yes, there's no denying that it fucks it up for a bit and, yes, it will almost definitely feel destroyed for a period of time after delivery, but it doesn't last forever. I can vouch for that with my own minge. Although it's definitely not as symmetrical as it used to be and my flaps are about 80 per cent droopier, when I can be arsed to actually have sex, it still feels as good as it did pre children. So don't let the gargantuan fanny fear hold you back, ladies, get your minge out and just give it a shot – how else will you know if you have a bucket or not until you test it out anyway?

Make nap-time naughty

Let's do this – all aboard the bone train. Woop woop! But wait a minute … you haven't even got to first base yet and there's a problem. What do you actually do with the kid? How do you tantalise a pair of testicles when there's a baby permanently attached to your tits? And if you do manage to find a moment together sans bambino, is it morally acceptable to be receiving a finger banging when said baby is under the same roof? And what if the rumbustious reverberation from your clapping cheeks wakes the baby up and they need feeding just as you're on the cusp of popping your socks? WHAT DO YOU DO?!

Chill the fuck out, babes. It's going to be OK. The brilliant thing about newborns is that they literally have no concept of what is going on. You can be as noisy and filthy as you like and even if you do disturb them, they won't judge you. They don't give a shit. Just choose a time when you know they're likely to sleep for at least thirty minutes or longer (you should be so lucky) and just bloody go for it. No hesitation; whip your knickers off, catapult yourself on to the captain and get your freak on. And if they do decide to wake up just as you're reaching the peak of pleasure, so what?! Either finish the job off as quickly and efficiently as possible or dismount, give yourself a wipe down and come back to the sex fest another day.

Let's get it on

OK, you no longer have the fear that your vagina will swallow your partner whole, the baby is fast asleep and you've just freshened up your flaps with a quick once over with your fanny flannel. Go pour yourself a glass of wine, whack on the Barry White and follow these tips to make this first sexual encounter post-birth the least awkward and most sensual experience you can possibly hope for.

Relax, baby

If ever there was a time to take a chill pill, it's now. I mean, don't go necking the Valium or anything, but if you're feeling tense or anxious about what's about to happen, do something together to unwind. This will help get you in the mood and keep you from tensing up and experiencing pain during sex. It sounds cheesy, but turning off the TV, putting on some music and sitting down to a candlelit dinner can really put you in the right frame of mind for minge. It may almost feel like a date! OK, so there's a baby monitor on the table and you have to pump your tits halfway through the meal, but we have to work with what we've got, people! Use this as an opportunity to reconnect with each other and, whatever you do, DO NOT TALK ABOUT THE BABY! Who am I kidding? What else have you got to talk about? But just try to keep the focus on each other and spend quality time together as a couple, not as parents. I guarantee that a couple of glasses of wine in and you'll be thrusting your genitals in each other's faces.

Warming up

Foreplay is integral during any sex session but even more so right now. You want to be well and truly warmed up before even contemplating penetration, as the more turned on you are, the more comfortable and hospitable your vagina will be. And come on, people, if my husband tried to enter my meat curtains after a 30-second kiss and a half-hearted nipple flick, it would be like trying to part two strips of freeze-dried beef jerky with a Pritt Stick. No thanks. You could offer your partner a massage (or rather request that they massage you) to kick-start proceedings and take your time to tease and tantalise one another with your fingers and tongues before progressing to the main attraction.

Slip and slide

Hopefully, plenty of foreplay will have you dripping like a leaky faucet, but the truth is, having kids can leave you with a foof that's drier than a cat's tongue. This is due to a drop in oestrogen levels after birth, that continue to stay low if you breastfeed. Oestrogen is important to sexual arousal because it boosts the flow of blood to the genitals and increases vaginal lubrication, so low oestrogen = arid minge. For those who don't breastfeed, your levels may return closer to normal within a few weeks of giving birth but the drought will continue for as long as you are nursing. Ensuring you have a well-oiled vessel makes for a much more pleasurable experience and prevents any potential fanny friction that may render penetration painful. Personally, I slather on the lube these days as a prerequisite to penile impalement. No grease on the pole, no entering my hole. So bulk-buy, bitches, you'll need it.

Your hole is not the goal

I know we've talked a lot about penetrative sex in this chapter, but remember, filling your hole doesn't necessarily have to be the ultimate goal. Sex encompasses a broad spectrum of pleasure, and if you don't feel ready for the full shebang, you can still enjoy each other's bodies and reach climax without committing to full penetration. Fact is, 75 per cent of women can't climax from penetration alone anyway, so it's the perfect excuse to ditch the dick and focus on your clitoris.

Ride it, cowgirl

As the first few times back in the sack are likely to be uncomfortable, experiment and find a position that doesn't aggravate your spam danglers and gives you control over the depth of penetration. You can try going on top but if you're a lazy bitch like me and can't be arsed to do all the work, try side to side. Doggy can do one. Just keep the thrusts slow and shallow and you'll be creaming your pie in no time.

Speak up to hot it up

Your partner can't read your mind or your minge, so lay out in explicit terms what you need them to do to get you off, and the areas to avoid if you're experiencing any discomfort down below. I know it can feel awkward vocalising what you want, but just imagine you're that chick off Google Maps and you have to audibly navigate your partner's journey through pleasure town. Turn left at the next junction, roadworks ahead, do a U-turn, take another left and Bob's your uncle, you have arrived at your destination!

The future is bright and full of boning

I hope you've finished reading this chapter feeling ready to whip out your whisker biscuit with confidence and sass. As we've discovered, sex is a complicated and nuanced business, comprising so much more than just physical attraction and lust. Your mind and body are intrinsically interconnected and if you're not in the right headspace for a boning, it's going to be shit. So be kind to yourself venturing back inside your vag, take your time, don't rush into anything because you feel you have to and only go back to it when you feel 100 per cent ready to ride.

It's easy to disconnect emotionally and physically from your partner when you are both focused solely on the baby, but once the newborn haze wears off and you regain a semblance of a life, you'll be able to reconnect like you once did. Saying that, I'm two years postpartum and I reckon I'd struggle to identify my husband's penis in a line up. These days I'm more likely to be deep-throating a tub of Ben & Jerry's than noshing off my husband. But do I care?! Sometimes, yes, but mostly, no! A monthly sex session is about all we manage to muster and we're both OK with that.

And remember, intimacy isn't just about exchanging bodily fluids. Emotional intimacy is just as, if not more, important than getting your end away. If there's an absence of emotional intimacy, one or both of you will feel a lack of love, support and overall connection. And no one has the inclination to get jiggy with a person they can't connect to. Taking the time to talk to one another at the end of each day, giving each other compliments or making a nice gesture, holding hands, cuddling, maybe even going in for a cheeky kiss – there are other ways to feel close and connected besides getting penetrated by a penis. All these little things add up to making you both feel secure and loved, which ultimately nurtures sexual desire.

So long as you are both open and honest about how you're feeling and neither one of you acts like a dick about it, you'll get back on track. And don't worry about the intercourse bit – sex is like riding a bike, sure, you'll need some oil on your rusty saddle but with a little practice you'll be back doing vaginal wheelies in no time.

14

LONELINESS

Marooned on the Island of Motherhood

As women, we are told that becoming a mother will fulfil us in ways we did not think possible, and that motherhood will enrich our lives with unparalleled levels of ovary-busting love, joy and connectivity. While it is true that many new mums do indeed experience these uterus-warming emotions, there is another significant byproduct of motherhood that appears to go completely unmentioned: loneliness.

It's ironic, is it not, that despite being attached at the tits to our babies 24/7, for most of us, our first prolonged experience of loneliness is felt during a time when we are rarely alone long enough to take a shit in peace. But it's the quality of company that counts, and there are only so many conversations you can have with an unresponsive ball of gurgling flesh before the grip of loneliness takes hold. Add that to the fact that your partner has probably gone back to work, your friends are busy living their lives, your own career is on hold, your family live miles away, plus you're dealing with all the emotional and mental turmoil that new parenthood throws up – physically and metaphorically – it's a sure-fire recipe for feeling isolated and alone. And if you're a single parent, it's even more debilitating.

There isn't much in-depth research on new parents and loneliness, but a UK survey of more than 2,000 mothers by the online mothers' networking group Channel Mums found that 90 per cent of mothers admit they feel lonely since having children and 54 per cent feel friendless after giving birth. For many, new motherhood can be so incredibly isolating that it leads to feelings of complete disconnect from the real world, like being shipwrecked from society and marooned on a faraway island. The Island of Motherhood. This feeling goes way beyond the baby blues and it's not a clinical condition, like postpartum depression (as we've previously explored), but instead it is a lingering sense of disorientation coupled with a loss of self. In fact, this tempestuous transition into motherhood has its very own term: it's called matrescence!

This chapter will explore matrescence and the expe-rience of loneliness in the first stages of motherhood, how it affects us, and what we can do to relieve it. From how to stop yourself going out of your mind with lone-liness on maternity leave, to tips for finding likeminded, wine-loving mum friends with whom to while away the time, right through to discovering how to keep the flame of your old self alight. Hopefully you will finish this chapter feeling more equipped to deal with your loneliness and realise that there are thousands of other lonely bitches out there who feel exactly like you. Because, sweetheart, you are not alone.

Matrescence – WTF is that then?

So what the hell is matrescence? Personally, I like to think of it as the mum equivalent of adolescence. Both signify a transitional phase of challenging change, characterised by surging hormones, bodily changes and shifts in your identity and relationships. And funnily enough, both also involve a fair amount of angst. But whereas adolescents get away with slamming doors and screaming 'I hate you' in the crux of their existential crisis, us poor matrescent bitches are expected to enjoy every second and be the happiest we've ever been.

You're probably wondering how this is related to feeling like a lonely cow. Well, while every woman's experience is unique, there are some universal aspects to the psychological narrative of matrescence that are very rarely acknowledged or discussed in an open and frank way. Feelings like ambivalence towards your children, mourning the loss of your identity and that old classic, mum guilt. Most of these thoughts and feelings are contrary to the belief that becoming a mother is the greatest gift we could ever ask for. They are kept secret out of fear of judgement and being ostracised by peers, family and, god forbid, other mums. So instead we repress these thoughts and let them fester away in our minds, feeling like we're the only ones who must think this way. And that's sure as hell going to make a gal feel lonely. Well, bullshit to that!

So where does this fear stem from? Why are mums across the globe literally 'keeping mum' about being mum? Surely sharing our experiences would lighten the mental load of motherhood and make us realise that we aren't alone in this parenting shitstorm. What are we so afraid of?

The 'Instagram' mum vs the 'hasn't washed her fanny in a week' mum

The idealisation of motherhood is everywhere in our culture. From advertising, press, TV, film and social media, motherhood is made to look like one big ovary jazzing, oxytocin-fuelled lovefest. It's enough to make anybody think that motherhood is easy. Social media is quite possibly the biggest culprit for perpetuating this myth as our feeds are filled with images of women who seem to effortlessly smash motherhood. Whether they are out at brunch, looking perfectly groomed with a cocktail in one hand and a serene breastfeeding baby in the other, or back doing yoga a week after giving birth, wearing Lycra leggings and not even a whiff of an engorged camel toe, these snapshots paint a picture of perfection, free from the struggles and challenges that most parents actually face. And meanwhile, you're scrolling through said photos while stuck on the sofa sitting on an ice pack for your haemorrhoids, with a cold cup of tea in one hand and a screaming baby in the other and all you can think is, 'How the fuck is she doing that?!'

Most of us are guilty of only ever sharing a highly curated slice of our lives publicly – it's the very nature of social media and unfortunately all it does is breed competitiveness and insecurity. There's rarely any mention of the shit bits; the brutal sleep deprivation, the endless hours cajoling a screaming baby, the fact your vagina may never feel quite the same again – oh no, you mustn't talk about that! You'll put people off having kids! Is it any surprise then, that when the reality of parenthood falls drastically short of our expectations, we feel that somehow we've personally fucked up. And then, added to that, no one else is admitting to finding it difficult too. That stuff makes you feel like you're a complete and utter failure and the only one in the world who isn't getting motherhood 'right'.

But it's an illusion, babes! There's no such thing as perfection. We don't know what's really going on behind that happy looking bint's skinny white jeans and freshly manicured nails. She could be miserable as sin, with piles just as angry as your throbbing anal grapes, but the difference is, she isn't choosing to share it! Well, lucky for you, I'm not that mum. I'm the warts and all, 'motherhood is bullshit', frank and honest bitch who talks about the tough stuff so you don't feel alone. So if you want to know what the majority of mums are really thinking but are too scared to admit, READ ON!

I love you, but you're a dickhead

Do you adore your baby but, equally, have moments of wanting to sling them in the bin? Do you relish hanging out with them, but can't wait for five minutes to yourself? Do you give them your everything but resent having nothing left for yourself? Do you love your role as a mum but simultaneously think motherhood is a big bag of flaccid dicks?

Of course you do, you're human! And pretty quickly these thoughts will pass and you'll be staring at your darling angels adoringly once more – although that only tends to happen when my kids finally fall asleep. Truth is, for most women, matrescence is one, long, complex emotional tug of war in which battling the push and pull of conflicting emotions underpins our very existence. One moment you think your kids are the best thing since sliced bread, the next they're little twats and you question why you ever had them. OK, that's a tad harsh (we've all been there) but ambivalence is a normal psychological reaction to the incredibly testing demands of parenthood.

In fact, ambivalence exists in almost all our interpersonal relationships to different degrees. Think about your partner, for example. Do you love them unreservedly 100 per cent of the time? Or are there moments when you want to throat punch them for eating a bag of crisps too loudly during a film or snoring like a cunt next to you in bed every night? Hell yes! We all have triggers that make us feel annoyed, resentful and sometimes even angry with the people in our lives, so why would it be any different with our kids?

But what kind of a mother resents her children? Errmm, every kind, Brenda, because contrary to the belief that mums shoot rainbows out of their fannies and love every second of wiping shitty arses, most of us, at some point, will find motherhood a complex, challenging journey to navigate. The problem is not the feeling of wanting to book a one-way flight to Rio and starting a new life without your family. The problem is the fear of speaking about it in the first place. That's what keeps us quiet, the judgement of others, so instead we cower alone in the shadow of shame and guilt feeling like we're the only one to have these thoughts.

But it's not true! Thinking your kids are twats doesn't make you a bad mum. I think it all the bloody time!

There are loads of us out there feeling exactly the same way, so how can we lessen the struggle? Well, what if we can learn to accept our own ambivalence, without trying to deny either the positive or the negative feelings? Things may be easier if we embrace the idea that we contain multitudes; and that feeling a mixture of opposing emotions is all part and parcel of the human experience, parent or not. We have to learn to sit in the middle of our love and our anger, our joy and our frustration, accept our feelings and know that loving our kids but also thinking they're little dickheads is perfectly normal.

Who am I?

Another key element of the matrescence period is grappling with the tension between your role as a mum yet still retaining a sense of your own identity. 'What's an identity?!' I hear the new mums cry. 'I think my personality fell out with my placenta!' It's true, the early stages of motherhood can leave you feeling completely bereft of your old self as your focus shifts from your own needs to those of your baby. You spent the last however many years defining your tastes, your desires, your ambitions, your intellect – all those factors that build up a complete picture of an individual – and then out pops a baby and it all just seems to fade into insignificance. Your purpose now is purely to provide for your offspring.

It's no surprise then that many of us feel lost in the midst of motherhood. In between the relentless pressures we face, the time devoted to caring for others, the lack of freedom and autonomy and then the expectation that mothers should devote their entire existence to motherhood, it doesn't feel like there's much room left for ourself. Even our bodies, still marred from the trauma of pregnancy and birth, feel alien and unlike our own. Of course that is going to trigger a confidence crisis and low self-esteem! Not only that, but how do you connect with other people when you feel like the discarded husk of your old, fun, interesting self? What are you even into now? Erm, coco melon? Bing? Mr Tumble? I DON'T FRIGGIN KNOW ANY MORE! Seeing old friends, making new friends, even relating to your partner can feel a challenge and, you guessed it, feed into the loneliness of matrescence.

It can be a frightening experience realising that you don't recognise yourself any more – not least because your tits now look like withered windsocks but also because you're too knackered to even remember what it was that once defined who you were. Well, don't panic, because despite the brain fog, the exhaustion, the general slog of the day-to-day mundanity of looking after kids, your identity is still there. When you become a mother, you do lose a part of your old self, it's inevitable, but the exciting bit of this is the opportunity that opens up for new parts of your identity to emerge and flourish.

Personally, motherhood has transformed who am I. Most liberating has been the gift of not giving a fuck any more and realising that other people's opinions of me do not matter – this from a girl who used to blush when her name was called out in the register. I'm wiser now, more emotionally resilient, less gullible and not afraid to fight for the things I believe in – and I put that down to motherhood testing me constantly beyond all my limitations. Sure, I can't hold my drink like I used to,

OK, I have to be in bed by 9p.m. and, yes, my vagina is 3cm wider than it used to be, but honestly, I love mum me more than I've ever loved myself before. All right, big head, pipe down!

Rather than thinking about it as a loss of identity, why don't we reframe motherhood as an evolution of our former selves. Is that not more empowering? Yes, we're mums, but we're also dynamic individuals with interests and passions that extend far beyond our babies. The two *can* happily co-exist. It's so important to prioritise yourself when you feel overwhelmed by the demands of motherhood and to share your experiences with others. As I keep reiterating, most women will have similar experiences as you and sharing that with each other is only ever going to make us feel less alone. And remember, taking time for yourself isn't selfish, and it doesn't make you a bad parent. I relish time on my own and having that break from being mum honestly gives me the space to reset and be a better parent when I'm with my children. And in fact, it sets an important example for your kids that their own health and wellbeing is of vital significance.

The mum guilt – will I ever be good enough?

So this leads nicely into our final segment of the matrescence period: THE MUM GUILT. Although, let's face it, guilt extends way beyond the initial stages of motherhood – this one is for the long term.

Now I was raised by a Catholic mother, so I'm no stranger to the concept of guilt and self-flagellation – in fact, it was a family fun activity! But there's something about growing a human in your uterus that seems to ignite a gut-wrenching penitence that overshadows every aspect of the mothering experience. And it starts the second that baby pops out of your minge.

From your feeding choices, your baby's sleeping arrangements, your parenting approach, leaving your baby with someone else, your ambivalence towards motherhood, when/if you return to work, your relationship ... need I go on? Nothing escapes the feeling of not doing enough, not doing things right or making decisions that may fuck up your kids in the long run. Sounds fun, right?!

But you're not alone in feeling the wrath of mum guilt. Research has shown that 87 per cent of mothers feel guilty at some point, with 21 per cent feeling this way most or all of the time. That's a dick load of women walking around carrying the weight of not feeling they're good enough. But is it any surprise with the external and internal pressures we all face: the picture-perfect depiction of motherhood on social media, the wildly high expectations from judgemental family, peers, other mothers and, above all, the scrutiny that we subject ourselves to?

The patriarchy of parenthood

Funny how there's never any reference to dad guilt, though. How come they get let off the hook? Are dads exempt from feeling parental guilt too? Of course not, but here's a thought: mum guilt actually serves an incredibly significant wider societal purpose. If women are the ones who are made to feel guilty, they will keep killing them-selves to do everything singlehandedly with very little support and never kick up a stink about it. We don't ask for the help that we rightly deserve because we're all striving to fulfil the ridiculous and impossible ideals of motherhood that are present in our culture. Admitting it's too much or too difficult makes us a 'failure', so we stay silent, which makes us complicit in a system that is designed to uphold the patriarchy. So I say let's fuck off this notion of 'mum' and let's just call it what it is; women being expected to nurture the next generation on their own so men can focus on more important things, like creating policies that discriminate against women and playing with their balls.

Personally, I've omitted guilt from my parenting reper-toire. Do I feel bad feeding my kids fish fingers three days in a row? NO! I just give them a bit of broccoli for balance. Do I feel sad leaving my kids to go to work? NO! I drop-kick them into nursery and skip into the sunset! Do I punish myself for hiding in the toilet for twenty minutes just to get some peace? NO! I take a book, a glass of wine and I make it a bloody event! I suggest you do the same too.

Let's not forget that the perfect mother shooting rainbows out of her minge is a myth. We're all just trying our hardest and our best, but the standards that society is setting for us are unreasonably high. And we are often doing this with little to no support. Guilt only serves to make us feel even more alone through this motherhood malarkey, so give yourself a break, love, drop your expectations and don't beat yourself up if you do something you later regret (like having kids in the first place). And most of all, take a look at your child – are they happy, clean, healthy, fed and loved? You can bet your bottom dollar they give zero shits about any of the stuff that keeps you up at night worrying that you're a terrible mother.

Keeping the loneliness at bay

No matter your circumstances or your support network, at some point we can all succumb to loneliness. And when those feelings of isolation arise, here are some tips to keep Lonely Larry at bay.

You do not have to love every second of motherhood. Some days are just shit and that's perfectly OK. Don't try to fight it, don't blame yourself for having a rubbish day and don't feel bad for wishing you could be anywhere else but stuck with your baby. Remember, you are only human and tomorrow is a new day.

Do something for you

Loneliness goes hand in hand with neglecting to look after yourself in the way you deserve to be looked after. Try to carve out time each day to do something for you, that reconnects you to yourself as opposed to something that focuses on your baby. Maybe that's sticking baby in front of CBeebies so you can do some exercise, having a tickle of your lady parts during nap time, or listening to a podcast while you push the pram around to get your stupid baby to sleep – little, achievable steps that take the focus off baby and back on to you. You need to remember that when you feel good about yourself, your baby will benefit. You are not being selfish if you take some time to care for yourself.

Get out of the house

Even if you just go for a walk, try to leave the confines of the four walls of your home each day. Fresh air and sunlight can do wonders for your mood and mental health, plus it opens up the possibility of interacting with other humans. Simple human contact can do a lot to alleviate negative feelings like loneliness and feeling overwhelmed – even when you're a hard-faced Londoner like me. Personally, my go-to baby activity was to visit one of the many retail parks around my area and indulge in some serious homeware perusal. It's amazing what a TK Maxx bargain purchase can do to help lift feelings of loneliness.

Ask for help from family and friends

If you're lucky enough to have family and friends nearby, lean on them for support. It's not a sign of weakness to ask for their help. Be honest, let them know what you're going through and allow them to get involved. Unfortunately, a lot of us don't have this help on hand, so make the most of it if you do.

Build your mum squad

We know the importance of finding your mum mates, and there is nothing more empowering than having a like-minded mum you can share your experiences with. Try to arrange a weekly meet-up, even if it's just for coffee or a walk round the park. Talking with other mums, having a laugh and just engaging in adult conversation can do wonders for alleviating loneliness. And if there's wine involved, even better.

Get online

Again, we've already delved into the power of the internet, so use it and get online. Find support groups and play-groups in your local area, and scroll through social media looking for other mums of your ilk. And, if you have a few best friends or family members that don't live nearby, the next best thing to seeing them in person can be video call-ing. Just seeing a loved one's face and having a conversation, even if it is over technology, can do wonders for lifting feelings of loneliness. And if you just can't get out of the house or you're not ready to join groups outside your home, using technology is the next best thing for providing human contact.

Talk to your doctor

If your loneliness just won't go away or if you feel depressed or anxious as well, talk to your doctor. It could be a sign of postpartum depression (see Chapter 9 for more details). If you act quickly at the first sign of a prob-lem, you can get the treatment and help you need right away. Don't be afraid to be completely honest about your feelings. Doctors see this kind of thing all the time and are there to help you. There is no shame in what you are thinking, feeling or experiencing.

Feeling bombarded by loneliness can impact even the most confident and self-assured mothers. The key is to not let it fester. Take small steps each day to connect with other adults and hopefully you will start to feel happier and more connected to the world around you. And remember, nothing is forever. This too shall pass.

A friend in need

So what can you do as a new mum to ensure that lone-liness doesn't take a debilitating hold? The solution seems fairly obvious: find some mum mates! Great! But how do I do that then? Meeting other parents in the early days of parenthood mainly comes in the form of baby groups and parent coffee mornings, but for many of us (myself included), it's actually pretty challenging to go on a networking spree when you're sleep-de-prived, your vagina is still held together by a thread and you're feeling like your personality is about as dazzling as a sloppy turd. Pregnancy is actually a much easier time to establish your mum squad as you still have the mental capacity to hold a conversation without forget-ting what you were saying halfway through a sentence.

It's so worthwhile putting some groundwork in before baby comes along, which means seeking out opportunities to bond with other preggos. Antenatal classes, hypnobirthing courses, pregnancy yoga – these are prime scenarios to bag yourself a mate or two. The benefit of meeting while pregnant is that you're all likely to be around a similar gestation, give or take a few weeks here or there. So when your babies are born they'll be around the same age, and you'll find you're facing the same newborn challenges together as opposed to alone. It's just nice to be able to WhatsApp someone during a 3a.m. feed and know that you're guaranteed a reply as they're also awake, sitting in the dark with their tits out feeding a baby.

But what if you missed the pregnancy friend-making boat and are now a lonely miserable bint stranded at home with your sprog? Well, it's never too late to make friends! Baby classes are prime pick-up joints for new chums, but expect your conversations to roll a little differently from normal adult interactions. There's rarely a, 'Hi, my name is Victoria. I like soul music, cooking, photography and the films of Stanley Kubrick.' Most parental introductions go a little more like this: 'How old is your baby? How was the birth? Is your baby sleeping?' Those are the three key questions that seem to always crop up, and before you know it, you're sharing the graphic details of your episiotomy and describing the state of your vagina to a complete stranger without even knowing their name.

But how do I know who to talk to? Everyone is busy with their babies and no one looks interested in having a conversation! And what if they don't like me or I don't like them? I feel like a plank. Unfortunately, it's not as simple as rocking up, making eye contact with the first bint you see and, hey presto, you're BFs for life. Friendship doesn't work like that, and finding like-minded people you get on with can be a challenge. But remember, somewhere in that crowd of mums there's likely to be at least one ally. You've just got to seek them out.

For me, humour has always been central to making connections with others and has played a major role in my quest to find mum mates. When I'm scoping out a potential friend, I tend to either drop a couple of fanny jokes into the conversation and see who laughs or look out for the mum who doesn't appear to be taking the baby class too seriously. Spot the only other person in the room trying to stifle their giggles at the ridiculousness of a group of grown adults waving streamers over their baby's faces and singing Old MacDonald – that's your person.

Of course, the whole friend-making process can feel a bit awkward, especially if you're a socially anxious twat like me, but honestly, just having a few people to meet up and have a chin wag with is so beneficial to your mental health and wellbeing. And look, these don't have to be the greatest friendships on Earth – we're not aiming for being the Thelma and Louise of maternity leave here. You just need someone who doesn't judge you, who you can have a laugh with and who won't report you to Social Services for calling your kid a dick-head.

And if the real world isn't offering up many opportunities to form friendships, let's not forget that there is also the wonder of the worldwide interweb at our fingertips. I know I ragged on social media earlier in this chapter, but for all its toxic shitness, there is also good. For me, Instagram has been a huge outlet during motherhood and kept me sane. When I began sharing my honest experiences of the challenges of motherhood, it amazed me how many other women said they felt the same way. What started off as a distraction from the boredom and loneliness of maternity leave quickly grew into a huge community of like-minded women who support and champion each other every single day. And you don't have to be the one posting about this stuff, just seeing other people's experiences that reflect your own can make you feel less alone.

It's helpful also to remember that your parenting life isn't going to end once you're through the matrescence period. We've got a lifetime ahead of this shit! If you don't meet someone immediately, there will be plenty of opportunities to engage with other parents down the line. This was certainly the case for me, and although I met some lovely, amazing women during pregnancy and in the early days of motherhood, it wasn't until Oliver was eighteen months old that my true kindred spirit mum walked into my life. And boy, what a difference has she made. Funny, honest, caring, supportive, loves a glass (bottle) of wine and is always there when I need her, she's the mum friend every woman needs.

You are not alone

I'm hoping this chapter has given you a better understanding of why so many women end up feeling alone and isolated during the matrescence period. It's pretty obvious where loneliness stems from when you break it down, but that doesn't lessen the pain of living through it and feeling completely disconnected from the rest of the world at a time when you need support the most.

If more people understood matrescence better, and knew that most people found it a challenge, that ambivalence was normal, that the reality of motherhood was miles away from what everyone expects it to be and that feeling this way was nothing to be ashamed of, then don't you think we'd all feel a little less alone? Damn right we would!

It's essential that we talk about these experiences and share a different perspective of motherhood that isn't Instagram perfect. Women need to hear that actually motherhood is fucking hard and the best way to do that is to say it out loud. My hope is that every mother will start sharing their matrescence stories without shame or fear and shout about the realities of motherhood with friends, family, at work, in the playground, to prospective parents and around the modern-day fire pit of social media. It's only together that we can debunk the idealisation of motherhood and make every mother out there feel less alone, feel less stigmatised, and know that she's doing a bloody brilliant job.

15

CONCLUSION

And so our journey through pregnancy, birth and the postpartum period reaches its digestive-biscuit nipple-shaped end. It's been emotional, people. Not least because writing this has thrown up so many memories of my own tumultuous foray into early motherhood that I've been reduced to ugly tears on more than one occasion. Even my postpartum bumgrapes have been affected and popped out to throb along in sympathy.

Having stumbled blindly through the postpartum period twice, I can safely say that there's no other experience quite like it. As the last fourteen chapters have demonstrated, it's a complex journey of physical, emotional and psychological transformation that happens at such speed and with such ferocity that it can leave you feeling like a startled rabbit in the headlights. And the incredible thing is that despite the utter chaos that ensues from extracting a baby out of your uterus, we keep on fucking doing it. Hundreds of thousands of women right now are in exactly the same position as you – whether struggling with horrific morning sickness, in the throes of having their cervix stretched out like pastry, pouring a jug of warm water on to their stitched-up perineum, sitting in the dark rocking a screaming baby, applying cabbage leaves to their ravaged nips or staring into the mirror thinking 'who the fuck is this person?' – some poor bitch has been in your shoes a million times over. Yet the bitter irony is that one of the most universal experiences, lived by billions of women all over the globe, can feel like the loneliest time of your life.

I want you to know that it does get easier. One day you'll wake up and the postpartum fog will feel like it's lifted. You'll probably still be surviving on broken sleep for a while, you won't be able to neck shots like you used to, and doing a jumping jack will nearly always end with damp knickers, but somehow you start to find little pieces of yourself again and claw back a new, albeit saggy titted, identity. Sure, there will always be challenges and new obstacles to overcome and your kids will probably continue to test you to your limit – but it's all OK. There are no hard-and-fast rules about how to raise children, and if people were more honest I think the majority of us would admit that we have no idea what we're doing. I know I certainly don't; I'm just working it all out as we go along, trying not to fuck up my kids or murder my husband, and I will continue to do so until I'm dead.

Because that's the thing about the parenting journey – there is never an end. It's for life, people! Even when your kids are old enough to call you a cunt and leave home, you're still responsible for the little twats. But that's for another book. Right now, your focus is surviving nine months of a swollen vulva, squeezing a giant cranium through your flaps and navigating the emotional rollercoaster that is the postpartum period. Easy breezy, right?

I really hope that the information shared over the last fourteen chapters alongside my own experience of becoming a mother has left you feeling somewhat more prepared and empowered to embrace the journey you've embarked on. No matter how many books you read (except this one) or how many people you talk to, I don't think anything can ever truly prepare us for the onslaught of parenthood. Of course, you can do your research and line up your support networks in advance, but until you're living through the chaos yourself, it's difficult to comprehend just how drastically motherhood changes everything.

So I'll leave you here, applying Anusol to the post-partum haemorrhoid protruding out of my undercrackers two and a half years after giving birth and wave you a fond farewell. Remember, motherhood is never as straightforward as being good or bad, it's an ever-evolving mix of the two punctuated by a series of the highest highs and the lowest lows. But no matter how challenging, how mind-bogglingly exhausting and how much of a massive headfuck motherhood really is, I hope that this book has proved that we're all in this shitshow together. Good luck on your journey and know that you're never alone. We've got this, bitches!

ACKNOWLEDGEMENTS

Thank you to the entire team at Harper Collins for having the faith in me to write this book, even when I didn't believe I could. Special thanks to my editors, Helen and Katya, for drawing the best out of me and embracing my overuse of the word fanny. And to my gorgeous agent Katie, who's forever working hard in the background to fight my corner.

To all the brilliant women in my life who have made my journey through motherhood that little bit easier. My long term BFFs Leanne and Hannah. Lannie, you're the funniest woman I know and forever cheering me up with your inappropriate voicenotes slagging your kids off. Ginge, Pat would be so proud of the mother you've become. Our Friday mornings together eating biscuits while we ignore our kids keep me sane. Jenna, you absolute slag, you'd be my bestie even without the kids. I don't know what I'd do without you. Laura, my BF in friendship and in business, you make me laugh until I piss myself and are always there no matter what. I feel so privileged to have you in my life and our weekly rants are my therapy.

To Laura, my incredible midwife, who I bonded with over a love of cushions and Ina May, and who heroically held my bulging perineum intact only two hours before jetting off on her holibobs to Spain. That's dedication! Thank you also for being the expert fanny consultant to this book. Massive thanks also to Anna, sleep consultant extraordinaire, who has helped my little ones but also provided her expertise in this book. And to Danielle, the tit wizard, for being an all round beautiful human being, helping women to lactate and casting her eye over this book.

To my brilliantly bonkers family. Mum, who aced raising four children and made it all look deceptively easy. You're the glue in the Emes clan and I honestly have no idea how you survived popping out and mothering so many tiny humans and have remained so sane and fashionable. And Dad, thank you for shaping my warped sense of humour with your wit and word play – even though you were never really there.

To all the mums out there who I've bonded with over the raw shitness of motherhood. Whether virtually or IRL, your support and solidarity mean more to me than you'll ever know.

And finally to my husband Rob. Without your support and sperm, none of this would have ever been possible. Thank you for grounding me throughout the madness of parenthood – I wouldn't want to be on this journey with anybody else. And to my darling puddings, Oliver and Edith. You are the loves of my life. I promise that any money I make out of this book will pay for your therapy when you're old enough to read it. Thanks for ruining my life in the best possible way xx